Equine Dermatology

Editors

ANTHONY A. YU
ROD A.W. ROSYCHUK

VETERINARY CLINICS OF NORTH AMERICA: EQUINE PRACTICE

www.vetequine.theclinics.com

Consulting Editor
A. SIMON TURNER

December 2013 • Volume 29 • Number 3

ELSEVIER

1600 John F. Kennedy Boulevard • Suite 1800 • Philadelphia, Pennsylvania, 19103-2899

http://www.vetequine.theclinics.com

VETERINARY CLINICS OF NORTH AMERICA: EQUINE PRACTICE Volume 29, Number 3
December 2013 ISSN 0749-0739, ISBN-13: 978-0-323-26134-0

Editor: Patrick Manley; p.manley@elsevier.com
Developmental Editor: Donald Mumford

Veterinary Clinics of North America: Equine Practice (ISSN 0749-0739) is published in April, August, and December by Elsevier Inc., 360 Park Avenue South, New York, NY 10010-1710. Business and Editorial Offices: 1600 John F. Kennedy Blvd., Suite 1800, Philadelphia, PA 19103-2899. Subscription prices are $270.00 per year (domestic individuals), $431.00 per year (domestic institutions), $130.00 per year (domestic students/residents), $315.00 per year (Canadian individuals), $543.00 per year (Canadian institutions), $365.00 per year (international individuals), $543.00 per year (international institutions), and $180.00 per year (international and Canadian students/residents). To receive student/resident rate, orders must be accompanied by name of affiliated institution, date of term, and the signature of program/residency coordinator on institution letterhead. Orders will be billed at individual rate until proof of status is received. Foreign air speed delivery is included in all *Clinics* subscription prices. All prices are subject to change without notice. **POSTMASTER:** Send address changes to *Veterinary Clinics of North America: Equine Practice*, 3251 Riverport Lane, Maryland Heights, MO 63043. Customer Service (orders, claims, online, change of address): Elsevier Health Sciences Division, Subscription Customer Service, 3251 Riverport Lane, Maryland Heights, MO 63043. Tel: 1-800-654-2452 (U.S. and Canada); 314-447-8871 (outside U.S. and Canada). Fax: 314-447-8029. E-mail: journalscustomer service-usa@elsevier.com (for print support); E-mail: journalsonlinesupport-usa@elsevier (for online support).

Reprints. For copies of 100 or more of articles in this publication, please contact the Commercial Reprints Department, Elsevier Inc., 360 Park Avenue South, New York, NY 10010-1710. Tel.: 212-633-3874; Fax: 212-633-3820; E-mail: reprints@elsevier.com.

Veterinary Clinics of North America: Equine Practice is covered in *MEDLINE/PubMed (Index Medicus), Excerpta Medica, Current Contents/Agriculture, Biology and Environmental Sciences,* and *ISI.*

Printed in the United States of America.

Contributors

CONSULTING EDITOR

A. SIMON TURNER, BVSc, MS, DVSc
Diplomate, American College of Veterinary Surgeons; Professor Emeritus, Department of
Clinical Sciences, College of Veterinary Medicine and Biomedical Sciences, Colorado
State University, Fort Collins, Colorado

EDITORS

ANTHONY A. YU, DVM, MS
Veterinary Dermatologist, Diplomate, American College of Veterinary Dermatology; Yu of
Guelph Veterinary Dermatology, Guelph Veterinary Specialty Hospital, Guelph, Ontario,
Canada

ROD A.W. ROSYCHUK, DVM
Diplomate, American College of Veterinary Internal Medicine; Department of Clinical
Sciences, College of Veterinary Medicine and Biomedical Sciences, Colorado State
University, Fort Collins, Colorado

AUTHORS

VERENA K. AFFOLTER, Dr. med vet., PhD
Diplomate, ECVP; Professor of Clinical Dermatopathology, Department of Pathology,
Microbiology, and Immunology, School of Veterinary Medicine, University of California,
Davis, California

KERSTIN E. BERGVALL, DVM
Diplomate, European College of Veterinary Dermatology; Assistant Professor, Department
of Veterinary Clinical Sciences, University of Agriculture, Uppsala, Sweden

VALERIE A. FADOK, DVM, PhD
Diplomate, American College of Veterinary Dermatology; Dermatology Department,
North Houston Veterinary Specialists, Spring, Texas

GUY C.M. GRINWIS, DVM, PhD
Spec. KNMvD, Veterinary Pathology, Assistant Professor of Veterinary Pathology,
Department of Pathobiology, Faculty of Veterinary Medicine, Utrecht University, Utrecht,
The Netherlands

SANDRA N. KOCH, DVM, MS
Associate Clinical Professor of Veterinary Dermatology, Department of Veterinary Clinical
Sciences, College of Veterinary Medicine, Veterinary Medical Center, University of
Minnesota, St Paul, Minnesota

LUIS M. LEMBCKE, DVM
Graduate PhD Student, Department of Comparative and Experimental Medicine, College of Veterinary Medicine, University of Tennessee, Knoxville, Tennessee

ROSANNA MARSELLA, DVM
Diplomate, American College of Veterinary Dermatology; Professor, Department of Dermatology, University of Florida College of Medicine, Gainesville, Florida

JEFFREY C. PHILLIPS, DVM, MSpVM, PhD
Diplomate, American College of Veterinary Internal Medicine; Assistant Dean of Research, College of Veterinary Medicine, Lincoln Memorial University, Harrogate, Tennessee

ANN RASHMIR-RAVEN, DVM, MS, PGCVE
Diplomate, American College of Veterinary Surgeons; Department of Large Animal Clinical Sciences Department, Veterinary Medical Center, College of Veterinary Medicine, Michigan State University, East Lansing, Michigan

WAYNE ROSENKRANTZ, DVM
Diplomate, American College of Veterinary Dermatology; Partner, Animal Dermatology Clinic, Tustin, California

ROD A.W. ROSYCHUK, DVM
Diplomate, American College of Veterinary Internal Medicine; Professor, Chief of Dermatology, Head of Specialty Services, Department of Clinical Sciences, Colorado State University, Fort Collins, Colorado

MARIANNE M. SLOET VAN OLDRUITENBORGH-OOSTERBAAN, DVM, PhD
Diplomate, ECEIM, Spec. KNMvD Equine Internal Medicine, Professor of Equine Internal Medicine, Department of Equine Sciences, Faculty of Veterinary Medicine, Utrecht University, Utrecht, The Netherlands

SHEILA M.F. TORRES, DVM, MS, PhD
Diplomate, American College of Veterinary Dermatology; Professor of Veterinary Dermatology, Department of Veterinary Clinical Sciences, College of Veterinary Medicine, Veterinary Medical Center, University of Minnesota, St Paul, Minnesota

J. SCOTT WEESE, DVM, DVSc
Diplomate, American College of Veterinary Internal Medicine; Department of Pathobiology, Ontario Veterinary College, University of Guelph, Guelph, Ontario, Canada

STEPHEN D. WHITE, DVM
Diplomate, American College of Veterinary Dermatology; Professor and Chief of Service Dermatology, Department of Medicine and Epidemiology, School of Veterinary Medicine, Veterinary Medical Teaching Hospital, University of California, Davis, California

ANTHONY A. YU, DVM, MS
Veterinary Dermatologist, Diplomate, American College of Veterinary Dermatology; Yu of Guelph Veterinary Dermatology, Guelph Veterinary Specialty Hospital, Guelph, Ontario, Canada

Contents

Horses develop many skin and respiratory disorders that have been attributed to allergy. These disorders include pruritic skin diseases, recurrent urticaria, allergic rhinoconjunctivitis, and reactive airway disease. Allergen-specific IgE has been detected in these horses, and allergen-specific immunotherapy is used to ameliorate clinical signs. The best understood atopic disease in horses is insect hypersensitivity, but the goal of effective treatment with allergen-specific immunotherapy remains elusive. In this review, updates in pathogenesis of allergic states and a brief mention of the new data on what is known in humans and dogs and how that relates to equine allergic disorders are discussed.

Allergies are common in horses. It is important to identify and correct as many factors as possible to control pruritus and make the patient comfortable. *Culicoides* hypersensitivity is a common component in allergic horses. The main treatment continues to be rigorous fly control and avoidance of insect bites. Environmental allergies are best addressed by early identification of the offending allergens and formulation of allergen-specific immunotherapy to decrease the need for rescue medications. Food allergy is best managed with food avoidance. Urticaria is one of the manifestations of allergic disease wherein detection of the triggering cause is essential for management.

Bacterial, dermatophilosis, and superficial ringworm infections are common skin diseases noted in equine dermatology. The ability to recognize and accurately diagnose the skin condition is key to selecting an appropriate and successful treatment regimen. Addressing underlying etiology, environmental management, and infection control play a crucial role in preventing relapse of clinical signs.

Equine Pastern Dermatitis (EPD) is not a single disease, but a cutaneous reaction pattern of the horse. EPD should be considered a syndrome, rather than a diagnosis. Uncovering the underlying etiology prior to treatment is key to minimizing treatment failures and frustration. To achieve a positive therapeutic outcome, treating the predisposing and perpetuating factors is just as important as addressing the primary cause of EPD. This article reviews clinical signs, differential diagnoses, diagnosis, and treatment of EPD.

Chronic progressive lymphedema is a disorder of many draft horse breeds that presents with progressive swelling of the distal portions of the legs. This is associated with scaling, marked dermal fibrosis, and the development of skin folds and nodules. There seems to be a genetic predisposition to altered elastin metabolism and impaired function of the lymphatic system in the distal extremities. Management is palliative and involves keeping the feathers clipped short, treating secondary infections, daily exercise and skin care, hydrotherapy, manual lymph drainage and compression bandaging.

Pemphigus foliaceus is the most common autoimmune skin disease in horses and is associated with the production of autoantibodies directed against surface proteins of the keratinocyte. Pemphigus vulgaris is a rare autoimmune skin disease in horses. Systemic lupus erythematosus and cutaneous lupus erythematosus are recognized in horses and both are rare. Bullous pemphigoid is a rare autoimmune disease in horses caused by immunologic attack of the basement membrane zone by autoantibodies. Erythema muliforme is an immunologic reaction in the skin in which keratinocyte cell death is the prominent change seen on biopsy. Purpura hemorrhagica is thought analogous to nonthrombocytopenic purpura in humans.

Equine sarcoidosis seems to be an emerging problem. As more horses are referred for dermatologic disease, equine sarcoidosis should be considered in any case of exfoliative and/or nodular skin disease with or without systemic involvement, including generalized granulomatous disease affecting most internal organs. Multiple breeds are affected with mares being predisposed. Affected horses are typically 3 years or older. The prognosis for generalized granulomatous disease is generally poor, whereas the prognosis for the localized cutaneous form is favorable but may require lifelong treatment.

Noninflammatory, nonpruritic alopecias are uncommonly encountered in the horse. Alopecia areata, an apparently autoimmune hair follicle bulbitis produces focal, multifocal to widespread hair loss. The skin is otherwise normal. Diseases that can mimic the widespread hair loss associated with alopecia areata include telogen and anagen effluvium, seasonal alo-pecias, follicular dysplasias (including color dilution alopecia), various nu-tritional deficiencies and chemical toxicosis, and diseases that result in defective hair shafts (eg, trichorrhexis nodosa and piedra). These prob-lems are differentiated by history, physical examination, trichography, and skin biopsy. Most are cosmetic diseases that do not have predictably effective therapies.

This article reviews various aspects of 3 clinical disorders associated with papillomavirus in horses commonly known as classical viral papillo-matosis, genital papillomas/papillomatosis, and aural plaques. Classical papillomatosis is usually asymptomatic and spontaneously resolves within 1 to 9 months; therefore, treatment is often not required. Genital papillomas/papillomatosis have not been reported to spontaneously re-solve, and there is increasing evidence that genital papillomas may evolve to in situ or invasive squamous cell carcinomas. Horses with aural plaques may be asymptomatic or may present with signs of ear and head hypersensitivity.

Sarcoids are the most common skin tumors seen in horses worldwide. The pathogenesis of sarcoids is multifactorial, including an association with bovine papillomavirus types 1 and 2 and a genetic susceptibility to tumor development. Clinical manifestations vary and include occult, verrucous, nodular, fibroblastic, mixed, and malignant (malevolent) types. The tumor is nonmetastasizing but can become very aggressive locally. Multiple tu-mors are common. All clinical types can be present in the same horse. No treatment protocol is universally effective. The tumor has a high risk of recurrence. Recurrent and large tumors are associated with poorer prognoses.

 Video of melanoma vaccine administration in horses accompanies this article

Melanomas are among the most common skin tumors in horses, with prevalence rates reaching as high as 80% in adult gray horses. Most mel-anocytic tumors are benign at initial presentation; however, if left un-treated, up to two-thirds can progress to overt malignant behavior. Standard local treatment options can be used to treat solitary early-stage lesions but do not address the underlying risk of recurrent tumor forma-tion or the transformation to a malignant phenotype. An understanding of the specific molecular genetic factors associated with tumor formation should lead to targeted therapies that can be used to treat or ideally prevent disease.

VETERINARY CLINICS OF
NORTH AMERICA: EQUINE PRACTICE

THE CLINICS ARE NOW AVAILABLE ONLINE!
Access your subscription at:
www.theclinics.com

Preface

Equine Dermatology

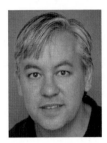 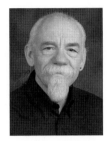

Anthony A. Yu, DVM, MS, DACVD   Rod A.W. Rosychuk, DVM, DACVIM

Editors

The last issue of *Veterinary Clinics of North America: Equine Practice* dedicated to dermatology was published in 1995. At that time, there were relatively few literature resources dedicated to the dermatologic diseases of horses. Since then, interest and expertise in equine dermatology has continued to grow. There are now several textbooks that provide excellent coverage of what has become a very lengthy list of equine dermatologic diseases. In this issue, we have not chosen to re-create a "mini" textbook. We have instead chosen to highlight a number of diseases or clinical presentations that we feel are clinically relevant, with a view to providing the most thorough and "up-to-date" information regarding their etiopathogenesis, diagnosis, and therapy. Commonly encountered diseases that are addressed include allergies (insect bite hypersensitivity, atopy, and food sensitivity), infectious diseases (staphylococcal infections, including methicillin-resistant *Staphylococcus aureus*, dermatophilosis, and dermatophytosis), equine pastern dermatitis, and sarcoids. Less common diseases are also discussed, both because they are still seen with some frequency in clinical practice and because there is significant "newer" information regarding their pathogenesis and/or therapy. These include papillomavirus-associated disease (classic papillomatosis, genital papillomas, aural plaques), melanoma, chronic progressive lymphedema, hereditary equine regional dermal asthenia, various autoimmune skin diseases (with emphasis on pemphigus foliaceus), sarcoidosis, and several nonpruritic, noninflammatory alopecic disorders (with emphasis on alopecia areata). Because donkeys have some unique features with regards to their dermatologic disease, there is an article dedicated to highlighting these differences. We are hoping to provide something for everyone. While busy practitioners may not wish to get bogged down in some of the esoterics of the cutting-edge concepts of etiopathogenesis that are discussed in some articles, you are strongly encouraged to visit the bottom-line therapeutic sections for these diseases, which contain the most contemporary, thorough, and complete information available. The authors that are contributing to this issue are leading clinicians in equine dermatology and researchers in the areas that they specifically

Vet Clin Equine 29 (2013) xi–xii
http://dx.doi.org/10.1016/j.cveq.2013.10.001
0749-0739/13/$ – see front matter © 2013 Published by Elsevier Inc.

vetequine.theclinics.com

address. We cannot thank them enough for their time and effort in providing the very latest information to all who are interested in equine dermatology.

Anthony A. Yu, DVM, MS, DACVD
Yu of Guelph Veterinary Dermatology
Guelph Veterinary Specialty Hospital
1460 Gordon Street South, Guelph
Ontario N1L 1C8, Canada

Rod A.W. Rosychuk, DVM, DACVIM
Department of Clinical Sciences
College of Veterinary Medicine and Biomedical Sciences
Colorado State University
300 West Drake
1678 Campus Delivery
Fort Collins, CO 80523-1678, USA

E-mail addresses:
yuvetpc@gmail.com (A.A. Yu)
Rod.Rosychuk@colostate.edu (R.A.W. Rosychuk)

Update on Equine Allergies

Valerie A. Fadok, DVM, PhD

KEYWORDS

- Insect bite hypersensitivity • Equine allergy testing • Food allergy • Atopy

KEY POINTS

- Horses develop several skin and respiratory disorders that have been attributed to allergy.
- These disorders include pruritic skin diseases, recurrent urticaria, allergic rhinoconjunctivitis, and reactive airway disease.
- Allergen-specific IgE has been detected in these horses, and allergen-specific immunotherapy is used to ameliorate clinical signs.
- The best understood atopic disease in horses is insect hypersensitivity, but the goal of effective treatment with allergen-specific immunotherapy remains elusive.
- The least understood is food allergy, for which there are very little hard data and no real feel for how best to diagnose it.

IMMUNOPATHOGENESIS

The term "atopy" describes an inherited predisposition to a constellation of diseases characterized by hyperreactivity to environmental allergens, including foods. These diseases in humans include allergic rhinitis and conjunctivitis, asthma, and atopic dermatitis. Production of immunoglobulin E (IgE) in response to the offending allergens is part of the disease process. The production of allergen-specific IgE is the basis of the intradermal skin testing and serum allergy testing and the findings have been used to generate allergen-specific immunotherapy with amelioration of clinical signs.[1–4] In the past, the production of IgE and its binding to the high-affinity Fc epsilon receptor on mast cells and basophils was the centerpiece of the understanding of atopy. Allergenic proteins were thought to be inhaled and somehow transported to the skin and mucous membranes, where they bound to and cross-linked cell-bound IgE. The rapid release of histamine and other preformed inflammatory mediators within minutes (type I hypersensitivity reaction) was followed by the later release of lipid mediators, such as leukotrienes and cytokines, that mediated inflammation (the late phase IgE response). Although it is known that these pathways occur, it has been learned that the

The author has nothing to disclose.

Dermatology Department, North Houston Veterinary Specialists, 1646 Spring Cypress Road #100, Spring, TX 77388, USA

E-mail address: vfadokdvm@nhvetspecialists.com

Vet Clin Equine 29 (2013) 541–550

http://dx.doi.org/10.1016/j.cveq.2013.08.005

0749-0739/13/$ – see front matter © 2013 Elsevier Inc. All rights reserved.

vetequine.theclinics.com

pathogenesis of atopic dermatitis in humans and dogs is much more complex, and this complexity is likely to be the case for horses too.

Most of what is known about atopic dermatitis has come from studies of the spontaneous human disease and experimental models in mice.[5–13] Many of the features described for the human disease have been verified in the canine disease as well, at least preliminarily.[14–17] The familial predisposition to atopy is associated with the potential inheritance of a large number of polymorphic genes that affect the function of the innate and acquired immune responses, as well as the structure and function of the skin barrier.[18,19] Abnormalities in the skin barrier are thought to allow for cutaneous absorption of allergenic proteins, which are taken up by dendritic cells and carried to the lymph node. Naive T lymphocytes are activated and, because the immune response is skewed toward a T-helper 2 response, IgE production is induced, and a variety of cytokines, including interleukin (IL)-4, IL-5, IL-6, IL-13, and IL-31, are released. IL-31, in particular, has garnered much interest recently because it can bind to receptors on neurons to stimulate itch. An eosinophilic inflammatory infiltrate and itch are significant features of the atopic response in the skin. Allergen-specific IgE binds not only to mast cells and basophils but also to Langerhans cells and other dendritic cells within the skin and mucous membranes and serves to capture allergen very efficiently. Subsequent exposure to the allergen results in amplification of the allergic response locally. Lack of suppression by T-regulatory cells is part of the disease process, although it is not clear whether decreased T-regulatory cell function is a cause or result of the disease process.

There is a complex interplay between the immune system and the nervous system, which promotes the sensation of itch.[10,20–23] Th2 cytokines, particularly IL-31, directly stimulate itch by binding to their receptors on nerve fibers. Other pruritogenic mediators, including histamine, proteases, substance P, opioids, neurotrophins, and other neuroactive peptides, enhance the itch. Secondary infections with Staphylococci and Malassezia yeast are frequent and further aggravate the level of itch in humans and dogs. It is thought that at least Staphylococci are involved in the impetiginization seen in horses. Much less is known about the role of Malassezia in equine atopic diseases, but the recent recognition of their role in cats suggests that mammals with atopic disease are more susceptible to these yeast infections and further work with horses is warranted. Inflammatory proteins from these microbes are absorbed more readily through the impaired skin barrier and contribute further to its breakdown. Staphylococci promote skewing toward the Th2 response, and many patients can develop IgE against bacterial and yeast proteins, resulting in bacterial and yeast hypersensitivity. Over time, as the disease becomes chronic, there is a shift toward the T-helper 1 cytokine response, with TNF-α playing a more prominent role.

It has been known for some time that the model of Th2/Th1 imbalance has been used to explain the immunologic abnormalities associated with respiratory allergies, but recent studies have shown that an epithelial barrier defect likely contributes to these diseases as well. Using biopsies from human patients with and without chronic rhinosinusitis, investigators measured trans-tissue resistance and found it to be reduced in samples from affected patients.[24] Furthermore, they showed that the components of tight junctions, occluden and zonula occudens 1, were patchy, irregular, and decreased in diseased tissue. By culturing respiratory epithelial cells in an air-liquid interface, these findings could be replicated in vitro. As well, addition of IFN-γ and IL-4 could mimic these changes when applied to epithelial cultures from normal individuals. Interestingly, a polymorphism in SPINK5 (serine protease inhibitor Kazal type 5) identified in human patients with atopic dermatitis has also been incriminated in human patients with asthma and chronic sinusitis.[19,25,26] This polymorphism is thought to be a marker for atopy in general. SPINK5 is expressed in all epithelial tissues and is thought to inhibit function of serine proteases. Another epithelial product central to atopy is the cytokine TSLP (thymic stromal lymphopoietin).[27] This cytokine is produced by damaged epithelial cells and it is known to induce the Th2 phenotype in atopic dermatitis, allergic rhinoconjunctivitis, and asthma. Equine TSLP has been cloned, and its RNA expression has been confirmed in the bronchoalvealar lavage fluid of horses with reactive airway disease.[28,29] Recombinant equine TSLP has been expressed, and anti-equine TSLP antibodies have been generated, which will allow for the study of this cytokine in equine allergic diseases.[30] In fact, single-nucleotide polymorphisms in TSLP have been observed in horses with insect bite hypersensitivity.[31]

It makes sense to hypothesize that mechanisms similar to those in humans and dogs mediate atopic diseases in horses, and evidence is slowly accumulating. The disease most like atopic dermatitis is the pruritus and dermatitis associated with Culicoides hypersensitivity and some horses with positive intradermal skin test or serum test reactions to environmental allergens. To call the disease atopic dermatitis, it must be verified that horses make IgE in response to environmental allergens, that they have an imbalance between Th2 and Th1 cells, that they absorb allergens through the skin, and that they have an impaired skin barrier. It is very clear that horses make IgE[32–38] and that allergen-specific IgE can be detected using intradermal skin testing and/or serum testing.[39–43] Based on what is known about mammalian IgE, it can be assumed that horses, like other allergic mammals, use the same immunologic mechanisms. Although evidence is lacking with regard to pollens, molds, dusts, or danders, there is good evidence that a Th2/Th1 imbalance is involved in horses with Culicoides hypersensitivity, and that this insect bite hypersensitivity shares many features with atopic dermatitis.

Heimann and colleagues[44] used immunohistochemical staining to compare the distribution of CD4+, CD8+, and FoxP3+ T-regulatory cells between normal horses and those with insect hypersensitivity. As would be predicted, there were increased numbers of T cells in the affected horses, but ratios of FoxP3+ T cells/CD4+ were significantly lower in affected horses compared with normal horses. Cytokine expression was assessed by real-time quantitative PCR. Affected horses showed elevated mRNA levels for IL-13 in lesional and nonlesional skin, and lower mRNA levels for IL-10 in lesional skin. These data could support the hypothesis that insect hypersensitivity in horses is associated with imbalances in the ratio of T-helper 2 cytokines and those produced by regulatory T cells. However, until the expression and function of the cytokine proteins have been demonstrated, no firm conclusions can be made.

Hamza and colleagues[45–47] took a different approach by culturing equine peripheral blood mononuclear cells in the presence of mitogen, insect allergens, or irrelevant allergens. The cells were subsequently examined by flow cytometry for cytokine protein production and total cytokine was measured by ELISA. There were seasonal differences in cytokine production from horses with insect hypersensitivity. Increased production of total IL-4, increased numbers of IL-4-producing cells, and decreased production of IFN-γ were seen in the summer, when lesions were active.[45] Subsequent studies showed that reduced incidence of insect hypersensitivity was associated with down-regulation of IL-4-producing cells and increased expression of IL-10 and TGF-β.[46] Equine peripheral blood mononuclear cells from affected Icelandic horses, when stimulated with Culicoides allergen, produced lower numbers of FoxP3+ T-regulatory cells than did those from healthy horses.[47] The addition of IL-4 to the cells of healthy horses was able to reduce the number of T-regulatory cells. These data suggested that the decrease in T-regulatory cells was secondary, rather than a primary cause of susceptibility to insect hypersensitivity. Last, as mentioned above, equine TSLP has been cloned, expressed, and antibodies against it developed, which will allow for study of the role of this cytokine in skin and respiratory allergies.[30]

Information about the genetic factors associated with insect hypersensitivities is slowly accumulating as well.[48] Differential gene expression in equine asthma is revealing potential new targets for therapy.[30,49] As these data accumulate, commonalities between horses and other animals with atopic disease should be discovered, and also interesting differences concerning the complex interplay between environment and genetics in allergic disease.

Barrier dysfunction is considered an integral part of the pathogenesis of atopic dermatitis. In fact, the skin barrier and the immune response are thought to be tightly linked.[50] Very little is known about the skin barrier of horses. An abstract recently presented at the World Congress of Veterinary Dermatology established that some of the ultrastructural changes associated with barrier defects in humans and dogs were seen in the skin of one atopic horse.[51] This finding supports continued study into the barrier function of horses, and whether barrier repair will become part of a multimodal approach to the management of atopic dermatitis in horses.

The role of food allergy in equine skin disease remains a mystery. Although food allergy is thought to occur, there is very little in peer-reviewed literature about its prevalence, its causes, or its pathogenesis. Anecdotal reports that chronic urticaria can be caused by food allergy suggests a role for IgE, but there is no hard evidence. Absolutely no information is available about the pathophysiology of food allergy in horses. Mechanisms mediating food allergy in humans can be humoral or cell-mediated. IgE-mediated disease results in the rapid onset of clinical signs after exposure to the food, whereas cellular mechanisms may have a more delayed onset. Food allergy manifestations in humans include urticaria and angioedema, but also eosinophilic esophagitis and gastroenteritis. Many of the mechanisms mediating atopic disease in skin and the respiratory tract have been demonstrated in the gut. Memory T cells specific for gut-associated allergens home preferentially to the gut on re-exposure[52] and dendritic cells have been shown to induce the Th2 response to food allergens.[53,54] Immunologic tolerance in the gut is actively mediated by regulatory T cells, which are induced by dendritic cells residing in the gut.[55] Experimental induction of food allergy requires genetic predisposition, adjuvants, and bypassing oral tolerance by exposure through other routes. These requirements are likely needed in the clinical disease as well; that is, disruption of the gut barrier by immunologic and nonimmunologic mechanisms, along with increased food allergen load, thereby setting the gut up for an allergic reaction.[56] Of interest is that newer evidence suggests that food allergy may be induced by exposure through a disrupted skin barrier and that early oral exposure actually leads to tolerance.[57] Because the gut microflora are thought to play a critical role in the establishment of oral tolerance, the use of probiotics has been studied and shown to have beneficial results in the management of food allergy.[58] The only reports of food allergy in peer-reviewed literature related to horses with recurrent urticaria are the implication that these are mediated by allergen-specific IgE.[59–61] Popular opinion suggests that pruritic skin disease might also have food allergy as a cause. The role of a Th2 helper response in equine food allergy remains to be determined.

CLINICAL DISEASE EXPRESSION, DIAGNOSIS, AND TREATMENT

Significant advances have not been seen in the diagnosis and treatment of allergic disorders in horses. Therefore a brief review of the diagnostic approach many veterinarians take with allergic horses follows.

EQUINE INSECT BITE HYPERSENSITIVITY

The most common equine allergy, and the best studied, is that to insects, in particular, Culicoides hypersensitivity.[62,63] This disease is characterized by pruritus and secondary lesions of alopecia and crusting. The distribution on the body is determined by the species of Culicoides feeding on the horse. The classic distribution is the dorsally distributed disease with lesions found on the face, mane, withers, rump, and tail ("sweet itch"). Ventrally feeding Culicoides spp cause lesions in the intermandibular space and on the ventral body wall. In some parts of the world, where there are several species of Culicoides, horses can have a combination of both. Furthermore, the species causing the disease may vary throughout the year, contributing to variation in distribution of clinical signs.[64,65]

The diagnosis of Culicoides hypersensitivity is made by history, clinical signs, response to insect control, and intradermal and/or ELISA testing (serology). An ectoparasiticidal trial for diagnosis can be difficult. These crepuscular insects feed at dawn and dusk and stabling the horses from dusk to dawn will help the problem. Fans can also be put into stalls so that feeding behavior is reduced, because these tiny flies are unable to fly and feed in brisk breezes. Ultimately, the regular application of insecticides is needed for control of this disease and permethrin seem to be the best choices.[66] Sprays are available but there are several spot-on treatments as well. Some veterinary dermatologists use the canine product Vectra 3D off-label for horses; this product contains dinotefuran, pyriproxifen (an insect growth regulator), and permethrin. Three tubes of the largest dog size are used: one applied to the mane and face, one to the back and rump, and one to the ventral abdomen. Testimonial evidence suggests that it is helpful but no published data are available.

Intradermal testing and ELISA serologic testing have been validated for this disease.[67–71]

Intradermal testing using Culiocoides extracts can be used as part of a complete panel to look at other allergic reactions. Progress has been made in identifying specific Culicoides proteins that induce immediate hypersensitivity in affected horses. In the Netherlands, 7 different proteins isolated from *Culicoides obsoletus* were used for ELISA and intradermal testing in horses.[68] This species was chosen because it is the primary species causing disease in the Netherlands. The ELISA reactions in affected horses varied from 38% to 67% depending on the individual allergen, but when all 7 proteins were used, there was a sensitivity of 92% and a specificity of 85%. These proteins were valuable in intradermal skin testing as well. When a protein from a different Culicoides spp (*C sonorensis*) was used in ELISA, IgE levels were lower. The conclusion was that for countries in which *C obsoletus* is the major parasite, these proteins could be useful for diagnosis and immunotherapy. It remains to be seen whether they would be useful for horses parasitized by other species. Similar studies using proteins from *Culicoides nubeculosis* have been performed in Switzerland.[72] Anderson and colleagues[73] in British Columbia demonstrated that immunotherapy can be effective. However, a placebo controlled study performed in Florida failed to show any benefit.[74] This clearly indicates that much more work needs to be done.

Horses can show hypersensitivity reactions to other insects as well, including blackfly, mosquito, stable fly, hornfly, and tabanids. These syndromes are less studied and most reports are anecdotal. Investigators have described allergens that cross-react between Culicoides and Simulium (black flies),[75,76] so it is possible that horses with Simulium allergies could benefit from Culicoides immunotherapy. Horses with Simulium hypersensitivity often have crusted pruritic papules where they have been bitten. Horses with Stomoxys (stable fly) hypersensitivity often have crusted pruritic papules on their chests and limbs. Mosquito bite hypersensitivity can be associated with generalized papular urticaria or true hives. Horses with Tabanid (horse fly; deer fly) allergies can have large ulcerated masses similar in clinical appearance to mild lesions of habronemiasis. Owners often report that the lesions develop where they see horse flies or deer flies feeding. It can be quite difficult to differentiate among the various insect hypersensitivities and it is likely that some horses are allergic to multiple biting insects.

ATOPY/ATOPIC DERMATITIS

A variety of syndromes have been associated with environmental allergies in horses including pruritus, similar to that seen with insect hypersensitivities, recurrent urticaria, reactive airway disease/chronic obstructive pulmonary disease, and syndromes such as head tossing and laminitis. Some of the pruritic horses may have combined insect hypersensitivity and reactions to pollens, molds, dusts, danders, or mites.

Diagnosis can be made by intradermal testing and/or serum allergy testing. There is some support in the literature for intradermal testing but very little for serum testing.[2,4,40–43] As for dogs, intradermal testing is not standardized for horses, which accounts for the variability in our literature. Serum testing offers increased accessibility to allergy testing for horses, and if the equine testing has improved as much as the canine testing has over the last 20 years, it seems reasonable to recommend its use, as most horses will not have the opportunity to have intradermal testing.

EQUINE FOOD ALLERGY

Very little is known about food allergy in horses. All reports are anecdotal and few reports are in refereed journals.[58–61] Reported signs include recurrent urticarial, pruritic skin disease, and anal pruritus. Incriminated foods have included sweet feed, oats, corn, other grains, dry garlic, and alfalfa. Diet trials in horses are difficult. The general recommendations are to analyze what is being fed and switch to a different grain, or drop the grain entirely for the period of the diet trial. The optimal length of time for a diet trial in horses is not known. It makes sense, though, that if the clinical signs subside with a diet trial, to prove food reactivity by challenge.

SUMMARY

The understanding of allergic disease in horses is lagging behind that of dogs, but progress is being made, particularly in the area of insect hypersensitivity. It is hoped that more effective tools will be acquired for the diagnosis and treatment in the foreseeable future.

REFERENCES

1. Tallarico NJ, Tallarico CM. Results of intradermal allergy testing and treatment by hyposensitization of 53 horses with chronic obstructive pulmonary disease, urticaria, headshaking, and/or reactive airway disease. J Vet Allergy Clin Immunol 1998;6:25–35.
2. Rees CA. Response to immunotherapy in six related horses with urticaria secondary to atopy. J Am Vet Med Assoc 2001;218(5):753–5.
3. Loewenstein C, Mueller ,RS. A review of allergen-specific immunotherapy in human and veterinary medicine. Vet Dermatol 2009;20(2):84–98.
4. Stepnik CT, Outerbridge CA, White SD, et al. Equine atopic skin disease and response to allergen-specific immunotherapy: a retrospective study at the university of california-davis (1991-2008). Vet Dermatol 2012;23(1):29–35.

5. Novak N, Leung DY. Advances in atopic dermatitis. Curr Opin Immunol 2011; 23(6):778–83.
6. Moniaga CS, Kabashima K. Filaggrin in atopic dermatitis: flaky tail mice as a novel model for developing drug targets in atopic dermatitis. Inflamm Allergy Drug Targets 2011;10(6):477–85.
7. Simon D, Kernland Lang K. Atopic dermatitis: from new pathogenic insights toward a barrier-restoring and anti-inflammatory therapy. Curr Opin Pediatr 2011; 23(6):647–52.
8. Rahman S, Collins M, Williams CM, et al. The pathology and immunology of atopic dermatitis. Inflamm Allergy Drug Targets 2011;10(6):486–96.
9. Boguniewicz M, Leung DY. Atopic dermatitis: a disease of altered skin barrier and immune dysregulation. Immunol Rev 2011;242(1):233–46.
10. Tanaka A, Matsuda H. Evaluation of itch by using NC/NgaTnd mice: a model of human atopic dermatitis. J Biomed Biotechnol 2011;2011:790436.
11. Takeda K, Gelfand EW. Mouse models of allergic diseases. Curr Opin Immunol 2009;21(6):660–5.
12. Jin H, He R, Oyoshi M, et al. Animal models of atopic dermatitis. J Invest Dermatol 2009;129(1):31–40.
13. Scharschmidt TC, Segre JA. Modeling atopic dermatitis with increasingly complex mouse models. J Invest Dermatol 2008;128(5):1061–4.
14. Marsella R, Sousa CA, Gonzales AJ, et al. Current understanding of the pathophysiologic mechanisms of canine atopic dermatitis. J Am Vet Med Assoc 2012; 241(2):194–207.
15. Olivry T. Is the skin barrier abnormal in dogs with atopic dermatitis? Vet Immunol Immunopathol 2011;144(1–2):11–6.
16. Marsella R, Olivry T, Carlotti DN, International Task Force on Canine Atopic Dermatitis. Current evidence of skin barrier dysfunction in human and canine atopic dermatitis. Vet Dermatol 2011;22(3):239–48.
17. Marsella R, Girolomoni G. Canine models of atopic dermatitis: a useful tool with untapped potential. J Invest Dermatol 2009;129(10):2351–7.
18. Grammatikos AP. The genetic and environmental basis of atopic diseases. Ann Med 2008;40(7):482–95.
19. Brown SJ, McLean WH. Eczema genetics: current state of knowledge and future goals. J Invest Dermatol 2009;129(3):543–52.
20. Suárez AL, Feramisco JD, Koo J, et al. Psychoneuroimmunology of psychological stress and atopic dermatitis: pathophysiologic and therapeutic updates. Acta Derm Venereol 2012;92(1):7–15.
21. Hong J, Buddenkotte J, Berger TG, et al. Management of itch in atopic dermatitis. Semin Cutan Med Surg 2011;30(2):71–86.
22. Lee CH, Yu HS. Biomarkers for itch and disease severity in atopic dermatitis. Curr Probl Dermatol 2011;41:136–48.
23. Darsow U, Pfab F, Valet M, et al. Pruritus and atopic dermatitis. Clin Rev Allergy Immunol 2011;41(3):237–44.
24. Soyka MB, Wawrzyniak P, Eiwegger T, et al. Defective epithelial barrier in chronic rhinosinusitis: the regulation of tight junctions by IFN-γ and IL-4. J Allergy Clin Immunol 2012;130(5):1087–96.
25. Liu Q, Xia Y, Zhang W, et al. A functional polymorphism in the SPINK5 gene is associated with asthma in a Chinese Han population. BMC Med Genet 2009;10:59.
26. Zhao LP, Di Z, Zhang L, et al. Association of SPINK5 gene polymorphisms with atopic dermatitis in northeast china. J Eur Acad Dermatol Venereol 2012;26(5): 572–7.

27. Ito T, Liu YJ, Arima K. Cellular and molecular mechanisms of TSLP function in human allergic disorders–TLSP programs the "th2 code" in dendritic cells. Allergol Int 2012;61(1):35–43.

28. Klukowska-Rötzler J, Marti E, Bugno M, et al. Molecular cloning and characterization of equine thymic stromal lymphopoietin. Vet Immunol Immunopathol 2010;136(3–4):346–9.

29. Klukowska-Rötzler J, Marti E, Lavoie JP, et al. Expression of thymic stromal 1lymphopoietin in equine recurrent airway obstruction. Vet Immunol Immunopathol 2012;146(1):46–52.

30. Janda J, Plattet P, Torsteinsdottir S, et al. Generation of equine TSLP-specific antibodies and their use for detection of TSLP produced by equine keratinocytes and leukocytes. Vet Immunol Immunopathol 2012;147(3–4):180–6.

31. Klumplerova M, Vychodilova L, Bobrova O, et al. Major histocompatibility complex and other allergy-related candidate genes associated with insect bite hypersensitivity in Icelandic horses. Mol Biol Rep 2013;40(4):3333–40.

32. Suter M, Fey H. Isolation and characterization of equine IgE. Zentralbl Veterinarmed B 1981;28(5):414–20.

33. Matthews AG, Imlah P, McPherson EA. A reagin-like antibody in horse serum: 1. Occurrence and some biological properties. Vet Res Commun 1983;6(1):13–23.

34. Suter M, Fey H. Further purification and characterisation of horse IgE. Vet Immunol Immunopathol 1983;4(5–6):545–53.

35. Marti E, Peveri P, Griot-Wenk M, et al. Chicken antibodies to a recombinant fragment of the equine immunoglobulin epsilon heavy-chain recognising native horse IgE. Vet Immunol Immunopathol 1997;59(3–4):253–70.

36. Wagner B, Radbruch A, Rohwer J, et al. Monoclonal anti-equine IgE antibodies with specificity for different epitopes on the immunoglobulin heavy chain of native IgE. Vet Immunol Immunopathol 2003;92(1–2):45–60.

37. Wagner B, Miller WH, Morgan EE, et al. IgE and IgG antibodies in skin allergy of the horse. Vet Res 2006;37(6):813–25.

38. Wagner B. IgE in horses: occurrence in health and disease. Vet Immunol Immunopathol 2009;132(1):21–30.

39. Lorch G, Hillier A, Kwochka KW, et al. Results of intradermal tests in horses without atopy and horses with atopic dermatitis or recurrent urticaria. Am J Vet Res 2001;62(7):1051–9.

40. Lorch G, Hillier A, Kwochka KW, et al. Comparison of immediate intradermal test reactivity with serum IgE quantitation by use of a radioallergosorbent test and two ELISA in horses with and without atopy. J Am Vet Med Assoc 2001;218(8):1314–22.

41. Kalina WV, Pettigrew HD, Gershwin LJ. IgE ELISA using antisera derived from epsilon chain antigenic peptides detects allergen-specific IgE in allergic horses. Vet Immunol Immunopathol 2003;92(3–4):137–47.

42. Morgan EE, Miller WH, Wagner B. A comparison of intradermal testing and detection of allergen-specific immunoglobulin E in serum by enzyme-linked immunosorbent assay in horses affected with skin hypersensitivity. Vet Immunol Immunopathol 2007;120(3–4):160–7.

43. Petersen A, Schott HC. Effects of dexamethasone and hydroxyzine treatment on intradermal testing and allergen-specific IgE serum testing results in horses. Vet Dermatol 2009;20(5–6):615–22.

44. Heimann M, Janda J, Sigurdardottir OG, et al. Skin-infiltrating T cells and cytokine expression in Icelandic horses affected with insect bite hypersensitivity: a

possible role for regulatory T cells. Vet Immunol Immunopathol 2011;140(1–2): 63–74.

45. Hamza E, Doherr MG, Bertoni G, et al. Modulation of allergy incidence in icelandic horses is associated with a change in il-4-producing T cells. Int Arch Allergy Immunol 2007;144(4):325–37.

46. Hamza E, Wagner B, Jungi TW, et al. Reduced incidence of insect-bite hypersensitivity in Icelandic horses is associated with a down-regulation of interleukin-4 by interleukin-10 and transforming growth factor-beta1. Vet Immunol Immunopathol 2008;122(1–2):65–75.

47. Hamza E, Steinbach F, Marti E. CD4(+)CD25(+) T cells expressing FoxP3 in icelandic horses affected with insect bite hypersensitivity. Vet Immunol Immunopathol 2012;148(1–2):139–44.

48. Andersson LS, Swinburne JE, Meadows JR, et al. The same ELA class II risk factors confer equine insect bite hypersensitivity in two distinct populations. Immunogenetics 2012;64(3):201–8.

49. Lavoie JP, Lefebvre-Lavoie J, Leclere M, et al. Profiling of differentially expressed genes using suppression subtractive hybridization in an equine model of chronic asthma. PLoS One 2012;7(1):e29440.

50. De Benedetto A, Kubo A, Beck LA. Skin barrier disruption: a requirement for allergen sensitization? J Invest Dermatol 2012;132(3 Pt 2):949–63.

51. Marsella R, Samuelson D, Johnson C, et al. Pilot investigation on skin barrier in equine atopic dermatitis: observations on electron microscopy and measurements of transepidermal water loss. Vet Dermatol 2012;23(S1):77.

52. Islam SA, Luster AD. T cell homing to epithelial barriers in allergic disease. Nat Med 2012;18(5):705–15.

53. Ruiter B, Shreffler WG. The role of dendritic cells in food allergy. J Allergy Clin Immunol 2012;129(4):921–8.

54. Kim JS, Sampson HA. Food allergy: a glimpse into the inner workings of gut immunology. Curr Opin Gastroenterol 2012;28(2):99–103.

55. Berin MC. Mechanisms of allergic sensitization to foods: bypassing immune tolerance pathways. Immunol Allergy Clin North Am 2012;32(1):1–10.

56. Kunisawa J, Kiyono H. Aberrant interaction of the gut immune system with environmental factors in the development of food allergies. Curr Allergy Asthma Rep 2010;10(3):215–21.

57. Gigante G, Tortora A, Ianiro G, et al. Role of gut microbiota in food tolerance and allergies. Dig Dis 2011;29(6):540–9.

58. Miyazawa K, Ito M, Ohsaki K. An equine case of urticaria associated with dry garlic feeding. J Vet Med Sci 1991;53(4):747–8.

59. Hallebeek AJ, Sloet van Oldruitenborgh-Oosterbaan MM. 'Oat bumps' in horses. Differential diagnosis and nutritional aspects. Tijdschr Diergeneeskd 1995; 120(20):588–91 [in Dutch].

60. Francqueville M, Sabbah A. Chronic urticaria in sports horses. Allerg Immunol (Paris) 1999;31(6):212–3 [in French].

61. Volland-Francqueville M, Sabbah A. Recurrent or chronic urticaria in thoroughbred race-horses: clinical observations. Eur Ann Allergy Clin Immunol 2004; 36(1):9–12 [in French].

62. Baker KP, Quinn PJ. A report on clinical aspects and histopathology of sweet itch. Equine Vet J 1978;10(4):243–8.

63. Schaffartzik A, Hamza E, Janda J, et al. Equine insect bite hypersensitivity: what do we know? Vet Immunol Immunopathol 2012;147(3–4):113–26.

64. Greiner EC. Entomologic evaluation of insect hypersensitivity. Vet Clin North Am Equine Pract 1995;11(1):29–41.
65. Greiner EC, Fadok VF, Rabin EB. Equine Culicoides hypersensitivity in Florida: biting midges aspirated from horses. Med Vet Entomol 1990;4(4):375–81.
66. de Raat IJ, van den Boom R, van Poppel M, et al. The effect of a topical insecticide containing permethrin on the number of Culicoides midges caught near horses with and without insect bite hypersensitivity in the Netherlands. Tijdschr Diergeneeskd 2008;133(20):838–42.
67. Peeters LM, Janssens S, Goddeeris BM, et al. Evaluation of an IgE ELISA with Culicoides spp. extracts and recombinant salivary antigens for diagnosis of insect bite hypersensitivity in Warmblood horses. Vet Dermatol 2009;20(5–6): 607–14.
68. van der Meide NM, Roders N, Sloet van Oldruitenborgh-Oosterbaan MM, et al. Cloning and expression of candidate allergens from Culicoides obsoletus for diagnosis of insect bite hypersensitivity in horses. Vet Immunol Immunopathol 2013;153(3–4):227–39.
69. Ferroglio E, Pregel P, Accossato A, et al. Equine culicoides hypersensitivity: evaluation of a skin test and of humoral response. J Vet Med A Physiol Pathol Clin Med 2006;53(1):30–3.
70. Fadok VA, Greiner EC. Equine insect hypersensitivity: skin test and biopsy results correlated with clinical data. Equine Vet J 1990;22(4):236–40.
71. Sloet van Oldruitenborgh-Oosterbaan MM, van Poppel M, de Raat IJ, et al. Intradermal testing of horses with and without insect bite hypersensitivity in The Netherlands using an extract of native Culicoides species. Vet Dermatol 2009; 20(5–6):607–14.
72. Schaffartzik A, Marti E, Torsteinsdottir S, et al. Selective cloning, characterization, and production of the Culicoides nubeculosus salivary gland allergen repertoire associated with equine insect bite hypersensitivity. Vet Immunol Immunopathol 2011;139(2–4):200–9.
73. Anderson GS, Belton P, Jahren E, et al. Immunotherapy trial for horses in British Columbia with Culicoides (Diptera:Ceratopogonidae) hypersensitivity. J Med Entomol 1996;33(3):458–66.
74. Barbet JL, Bevier D, Greiner EC. Specific immunotherapy in the treatment of Culicoides hypersensitive horses: a double-blind study. Equine Vet J 1990;22(4): 232–5.
75. Hellberg W, Mellor PS, Torsteinsdóttir S, et al. Insect bite hypersensitivity in the horse: comparison of IgE-binding proteins in salivary gland extracts from Simulium vittatum and Culicoides nubeculosus. Vet Immunol Immunopathol 2009; 132(1):62–7.
76. Schaffartzik A, Weichel M, Crameri R, et al. Cloning of IgE-binding proteins from Simulium vittatum and their potential significance as allergens for equine insect bite hypersensitivity. Vet Immunol Immunopathol 2009;132(1):68–77.

Equine Allergy Therapy
Update on the Treatment of Environmental, Insect Bite Hypersensitivity, and Food Allergies

Rosanna Marsella, DVM, DACVD

KEYWORDS

- Atopic dermatitis • *Culicoides* hypersensitivity • Environmental allergies
- Food-induced dermatitis • Urticaria

KEY POINTS

- Allergies are extremely common in horses and may represent a diagnostic and therapeutic challenge for practitioners.
- As allergies are multifactorial and additive, it is important to identify and correct as many factors as possible to control pruritus and make the patient comfortable.
- *Culicoides* hypersensitivity is a common component in allergic horses, but despite significant advances in the understanding of the pathogenesis of the disease, the main treatment continues to be rigorous fly control and avoidance of insect bites.
- Environmental allergies are best addressed by early identification of the offending allergens and formulation of allergen-specific immunotherapy to decrease the need for rescue medications.
- Food allergy, diagnosed with a food trial followed by rechallenge, is best managed with food avoidance.

GENERAL CONCEPTS FOR THE MANAGEMENT OF ALLERGIC HORSES

Therapy of allergic diseases is closely linked to the diagnostic approach to the pruritic horse, as management of allergic cases requires a process of elimination of offending causes. Allergies are multifactorial and additive. Most patients have multiple allergies, and it is crucial to properly identify all the factors that contribute to the clinical signs in each patient in order to successfully control them. Many of these patients are atopic and therefore are prone to develop an allergic response to many different allergens ranging from pollens to insects, and sometimes also foods. As pruritus develops, self-trauma is common, and that frequently leads to secondary infections. Thus,

The author has nothing to disclose.
Department of Dermatology, University of Florida College of Medicine, PO Box 100126, Gainesville, FL 32610-0126, USA
E-mail address: marsella@ufl.edu

Vet Clin Equine 29 (2013) 551–557
http://dx.doi.org/10.1016/j.cveq.2013.08.006   **vetequine.theclinics.com**

management of these cases requires identification and correction of all factors playing a role in the level of pruritus. According to the theory of the pruritic threshold, an individual is able to tolerate a certain amount of pruritic stimuli without developing clinical signs. Once that threshold is exceeded, clinical signs ensue. Thus a large part of the management of these cases involves identifying that pruritic threshold and removing or correcting as many factors as possible in order to take the patient below the pruritic threshold (**Fig. 1**).

CULICOIDES HYPERSENSITIVITY

Although much progress has been made in the understanding of the pathogenesis of *Culicoides* hypersensitivity, the treatment for this condition is still unsatisfactory.[1] Management of *Culicoides* hypersensitivity can be summarized in 3 points:

1. Control the itch to prevent additional self-trauma.
2. Resolve secondary infections.
3. Prevent additional bites.

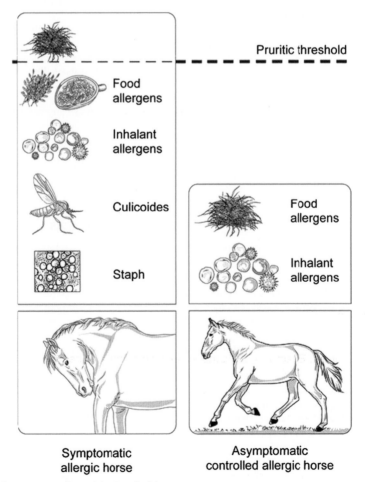

Fig. 1. The concept of pruritic threshold.

Control of the Itch

Control of the itch typically involves a combination of topical and systemic glucocorticoids depending on the severity of the clinical signs. It is always preferred to use topical therapy when possible to minimize the use of systemic glucocorticoids and decrease the risk for laminitis. Topical glucocorticoid therapy can be accomplished by using topical triamcinolone spray and a leave-on hydrocortisone conditioner. There are also a variety of glucocorticoid shampoos and lotions containing ingredients such as fluocinolone acetonide that can be used. When using shampoo therapy, it is recommended that the shampoo be left on the skin for 10 minutes before rinsing to maximize contact time and increase the efficacy of topical therapy. Lotions are particularly helpful for therapy of localized lesions such as the face and ears, which are not amenable to shampoo therapy. For more severe cases, prednisolone can be used systemically at an induction dose of 2 mg/kg every 24 hours for 3 to 10 days. Once the pruritus is controlled, this dose can be tapered to 0.5 mg/kg every 48 hours. Some horses may require dexamethasone (0.2 mg/kg every 24 hours), although this is not recommended for long-term management.

Antihistamines are another nonglucocorticoid alternative to decrease pruritus, although therapeutic success appears to be limited. Few published studies exist on the efficacy of antihistamines in horses with allergic disease. A recently published study reported no benefit with the use of cetirizine in horses with insect hypersensitivity.[2] Other antihistamines commonly prescribed include hydroxyzine (1–2 mg/kg every 8–12 hours by mouth) and chlorpheniramine (0.25–0.5 mg/kg every 12 hours by mouth). It is important to note that antihistamines seem to work best as a preventative before the beginning of allergy season and much less once the season has started. If needed, they can be combined with glucocorticoids. It is the clinical impression of the author that antihistamines appear to work best in combination with other allergy therapies and in patients with an environmental allergy rather than in horses that primarily suffer from *Culicoides* hypersensitivity.

Another treatment option to help decrease the need for glucocorticoids is the use of fatty acid supplementation, although efficacy is limited. A supplement containing sunflower oil, vitamins, amino acids, and peptides was tested in a controlled double-blinded clinical trial, but no significant differences in treatment-groups were noted when symptom severity was scored by the horse owners.[3] Flax seed has been used to decrease inflammation in allergic horses.[4] This supplement is well tolerated and may help to decrease clinical signs.

Resolve Secondary Infections

This second point in the management of *Culicoides* hypersensitivity requires a combination of topical antimicrobial therapy and, for more severe cases, systemic antibiotics. Topical antimicrobial therapy can be accomplished with shampoos, sprays, and conditioners. Examples of shampoos include chlorhexidine-, benzoyl peroxide-, and ethyl lactate-containing products. Benzoyl peroxide is effective in removing crusts, but it may dry and bleach the coat in some animals. Ethyl lactate is an effective antimicrobial that appears gentler and less drying than other antimicrobial products. Examples of antimicrobial sprays include oxychlorine-based products and 0.4% stannous fluoride, which has been demonstrated to be an effective treatment for staphylococcal infection in horses.[5] In terms of systemic antibiotic therapy, potentiated sulfonamides are a common empiric choice for staphylococcal infections. In chronic cases that have already had multiple courses of antibiotics, it may be helpful to submit a culture to test for antibiotic resistance and base the treatment recommendation on these findings. The average case of bacterial folliculitis requires 3 weeks of oral antibiotics. One of the adverse effects of prolonged therapy with potentiated sulfonamides is colitis. Horses treated with this antibiotic will need to be monitored for diarrhea.

Prevent Additional Insect Bites

The third point in the management of *Culicoides* hypersensitive horses involves strategies to decrease the number of bites. This can be accomplished in a number of ways, ranging from the diligent daily use of insect repellents to stalling the affected horse in front of strong fans at times when are most active (dusk and dawn). To help minimize exposure to *Culicoides*, horses should be moved to paddocks further away from bodies of standing water where these gnats breed. Gnats do not fly a long distance from their breeding grounds and do not fly well against the wind.

In terms of insect repellents, many products are available on the market and are labeled as insect repellents. In reality, many of them are just insecticides and not true repellents. Preference should be given to products containing 2% or higher of permethrin in formulations that adhere to the coat and are not easily washed off by the rain. Many spot on formulations with 44% to 64% permethrin are available on the market for specific use in horses. At this high percentage, a good repellent activity is obtained. These products can be used on specific problem areas (pole, base of the tail, base of the neck) once weekly, while sprays with lower concentrations (2% permethrin) may be used to cover the rest of the body. Besides permethrin, other synthetic pyrethroids such as cypermethrin can be effective repellents. Regardless of the product used, frequent (in most cases daily) reapplication is key, because even the best product does not have a long residual efficacy when horses sweat or are in high-humidity climates. Fly masks and fly sheets may be used as long as they are changed frequently. Soiled coverings may predispose to secondary infections, especially if they trap moisture in the heat of the summer.

ATOPIC DERMATITIS

Environmental allergies are the second most common allergy seen in horses. Management of atopic dermatitis can be done both symptomatically, by suppressing the inflammation and the pruritus triggered by the allergic response, and by addressing the specific cause (ie, by identifying the responsible allergens and formulating an allergen-specific vaccine).

The symptomatic approach is typically needed in the short term to make the patient comfortable and minimize self-trauma. This approach relies on the use of a combination of topical and systemic therapies including antihistamines, essential fatty acids, pentoxifylline, and glucocorticoids. Mild cases may respond to a combination of antihistamines and essential fatty acids. This approach is aimed more at preventing or minimizing the severity of flare ups, rather than controlling acute, more severe flare ups, which may require more aggressive therapy with glucocorticoids. Pentoxifylline has been found to be beneficial in moderate cases of atopic dermatitis. This drug is typically well tolerated and is safe for long-term use. Occasionally sweats and irritability have been reported by owners. Pentoxifylline is commonly prescribed at the dose of 8 to 10 mg/kg every 8 to 12 hours.

The primary approach to environmental allergy control involves the identification of allergens that trigger the hypersensitivity reaction. Allergy testing is used to detect the presence of allergen-specific immunoglobulin E (IgE). It is important to note that allergy testing (either serology or intradermal skin testing) simply detects allergen-specific IgE; showing a positive reaction does not necessarily mean that the response is clinically relevant. Thus, it is important to correlate the positive reactions detected in the allergy test with the seasonality and the environment of the patient to increase the likelihood of formulating a vaccine that includes clinically relevant allergens for each specific patient.[6] Debate exists on which type of allergy testing is the best. It is important to recognize that these 2 tests measure different things. Serology testing measures circulating allergen-specific IgE, while intradermal skin testing detects cutaneous allergen-specific IgE. It is also important to note that different companies typically use different sources of allergens. These facts help explain why the correlation between various tests is typically not very good.[7] Fortunately, the single most important aspect in formulating a successful immunotherapy is not which test is used but how the allergens are selected (ie, emphasis is placed on correlating the results with the seasonality and environmental exposure of the individual patient to increase the likelihood of including clinically relevant allergens among the ones that tested positive).

It is commonly accepted by dermatologists that allergen-specific immunotherapy can be of help to atopic horses. Few controlled studies have been done to date. Reported success rates vary from 60% to 80%.[8–10] This clinical impression has been supported by a recently published retrospective study that documented owners' impression of response to allergen-specific Immunotherapy.[11] In this study, 84% of owners reported a good response. More specifically, 93% of owners reported having to use glucocorticoids before initiating allergen-specific immunotherapy, and after 1 year of therapy 59% of cases were managed with immunotherapy alone. There was no statistical difference between type of test and reported success of allergen-specific immunotherapy, emphasizing that the key to success of immunotherapy may not lay in the specific test used. As a general rule, most horses show improvement after the first 6 months of therapy and some even after the first 3 months. Immunotherapy should be continued for a full year to completely assess for benefit.

FOOD ALLERGY

Therapy of horses with food hypersensitivity requires avoidance. Currently, allergen-specific immunotherapy is only done for environmental allergens and has not been used for food allergy. Successful therapy therefore relies on the proper identification of the correct food trigger. This requires a food trial with rechallenge to demonstrate that worsening of clinical signs occurs after exposure to certain foods. Once this is done, these foods are strictly avoided in the main diet as well as in any flavored supplement given to the horse. Knowledge of labels of the various commercial diets is essential. Common problematic diet ingredients include hays rich in protein such as alfalfa or peanut. Soybean is also a frequent culprit. Potential exposure to this needs to be researched, as soybean is frequently included in commercially prepared feeds, making long-term management difficult when using these commercially prepared feeds.

CONTACT ALLERGY

Therapy for contact allergy also relies on identification of the offending allergen and by practicing avoidance. Contact allergy is a type 4 hypersensitivity and is not amenable to immunotherapy. Identification of the offending allergen can be done by isolation and rechallenge or, more specifically, done by patch testing. In the patch test, small amounts of suspected substances ranging from plants to shavings or even sprays are placed onto an area of skin 24 to 48 hours after shaving. These test allergens are kept under an occlusive patch for 24 to 48 hours. After this period of time, the patch is removed, and the reaction is evaluated over the following 24 to 48 hours. A positive reaction is indicated by erythema and a papular reaction at the site of application.

For cases in which patch testing or avoidance cannot be done, it is useful to try pentoxifylline. This drug has been shown to decrease the severity of contact allergy in humans, dogs, and rodents.[12–14] Although studies have not been done in horses, it seems to help horses with allergies, including contact allergy. Pentoxifylline is typically well tolerated, but it can be costly for long-term use. Severe cases may still require glucocorticoid therapy to decrease clinical signs with acute flare-ups. It is also important to note that shampoo therapy to wash off the allergen is an important part of therapy. Mild, moisturizing shampoos with oatmeal can be used to decrease pruritus and self-trauma.

URTICARIA

One of the many manifestations of allergies in horses is urticaria. The causes for chronic urticaria in horses are numerous. Part of the treatment of these frustrating cases emphasizes the identification and management of the triggering cause. For this reason, it is important to take a through history, including information about exposure to drugs, vaccines, dewormers, supplements, and feeds. In some cases, urticaria is triggered by cold temperature, water, exercise, physical trauma, or pressure. Some cases are related to insect hypersensitivity, and others have pollen allergies and/or food allergies.[15] When a cause cannot be identified, symptomatic treatment is the only option. In most cases this involves the long-term use of glucocorticoids, because antihistamines are typically of limited benefit. Of all antihistamines, hydroxyzine is probably the most helpful to try. Pentoxifylline should also be tried. This drug has been shown to stabilize mast cells in other species.[16]

SUMMARY

In summary, the treatment of allergies in horses requires a comprehensive approach to identify and correct all possible contributing factors. The clinician should therefore be aware of the various contributors to the pruritus of each specific case and attempt to either treat or control each of them. For individuals with long seasons of environmental allergies, immunotherapy remains the best long-term option.

REFERENCES

1. Schaffartzik A, Hamza E, Janda J, et al. Equine insect bite hypersensitivity: what do we know? Vet Immunol Immunopathol 2012;147(3–4):113–26.
2. Olsén L, Bondesson U, Broström H, et al. Pharmacokinetics and effects of cetirizine in horses with insect bite hypersensitivity. Vet J 2011;187(3):347–51.
3. van den Boom R, Driessen F, Streumer SJ, et al. The effect of a supplement containing sunflower oil, vitamins, amino acids, and peptides on the severity of symptoms in horses suffering insect bite hypersensitivity. Tijdschr Diergeneeskd 2010;135(13):520–5.
4. O'Neill W, McKee S, Clarke AF. Flaxseed (Linum usitatissimum) supplementation associated with reduced skin test lesional area in horses with Culicoides hypersensitivity. Can J Vet Res 2002;66(4):272–7.
5. Marsella R, Akucewich L. Investigation on the clinical efficacy and tolerability of a 0.4% topical stannous fluoride preparation (MedEquine Gel) for the treatment of

bacterial skin infections in horses: a prospective, randomized, double-blinded, placebo-controlled clinical trial. Vet Dermatol 2007;18(6):444–50.

6. Lorch G, Hillier A, Kwochka KW, et al. Results of intradermal tests in horses without atopy and horses with atopic dermatitis or recurrent urticaria. Am J Vet Res 2001;62(7):1051–9.

7. Lorch G, Hillier A, Kwochka KW, et al. Comparison of immediate intradermal test reactivity with serum IgE quantitation by use of a radioallergosorbent test and two ELISA in horses with and without atopy. J Am Vet Med Assoc 2001;218(8):1314–22.

8. Fadok VA. Hyposensitization of equids with allergic skin/pulmonary diseases. In: Proceedings of the Annual Meeting of the American Academy of Veterinary Dermatology and the American College of Veterinary Dermatology. 1996. p. 47.

9. Fadok VA. Overview of equine pruritus. Vet Clin North Am Equine Pract 1995; 11(1):1–10.

10. Rosenkrantz WS, Griffin CE. Treatment of equine urticaria and pruritus with hyposensitization and antihistamines. In: Proceedings of the Annual Meeting of the American Academy of Veterinary Dermatology and the American College of Veterinary Dermatology 1986. p. 33.

11. Stepnik CT, Outerbridge CA, White SD, et al. Equine atopic skin disease and response to allergen-specific immunotherapy: a retrospective study at the University of California-Davis (1991-2008). Vet Dermatol 2012;23(1):29–35.

12. Saricaoğlu H, Tunali S, Bülbül E, et al. Prevention of nickel-induced allergic contact reactions with pentoxifylline. Contact Derm 1998;39(5):244–7.

13. Schwarz A, Krone C, Trautinger F, et al. Pentoxifylline suppresses irritant and contact hypersensitivity reactions. J Invest Dermatol 1993;101(4):549–52.

14. Marsella R, Kunkle GA, Lewis DT. Pentoxifylline inhibits contact hypersensitivity reactions to plants of the Commelinceae family in dogs. Vet Dermatol 1997; 8(2):121–6.

15. Volland-Francqueville M, Sabbah A. Recurrent or chronic urticaria in thoroughbred race-horses: clinical observations. Eur Ann Allergy Clin Immunol 2004; 36(1):9–12.

16. Babaei S, Bayat M. Effect of pentoxifylline administration on mast cell numbers and degranulation in a diabetic and normoglycemic rat model wound healing. Iran Red Crescent Med J 2012;14(8):483–7.

Infectious Folliculitis and Dermatophytosis

J. Scott Weese, DVM, DVSc[a],*, Anthony A. Yu, DVM, MS[b]

KEYWORDS

- *Staphylococcus* • Methicillin-resistant *Staphylococcus aureus* • *Dermatophilus*
- Rainrot • Dermatophytosis • Ringworm

KEY POINTS

- Bacterial, dermatophilosis, and superficial ringworm infections are common skin diseases noted in equine dermatology.
- The ability to recognize and accurately diagnose the skin condition is key to selecting an appropriate and successful treatment regimen.
- Addressing underlying etiology, environmental management, and infection control play a crucial role in preventing relapse of clinical signs.

BACTERIAL FOLLICULITIS
Staphylococcal Folliculitis

Staphylococci are common components of the commensal microbiota of the skin and mucous membranes, but are also important opportunistic pathogens. A wide variety of staphylococcal species can be found in or on healthy horses, and these differ greatly in their clinical relevance. It is reasonable to assume that 1 or more staphylococci can be found in or on virtually every healthy horse, typically with no clinical impact. However, staphylococci are leading causes of opportunistic infections that arise secondary to breaches in the normal physical and immunologic protective mechanisms.

An area of particular concern with staphylococci is their tendency to become resistant to antimicrobials. In particular, the emergence of methicillin-resistant staphylococci has caused much concern for both animal health and zoonotic infection. Although methicillin-resistant staphylococci are not inherently more virulent than their susceptible counterparts, they may be difficult to treat, outbreaks may occur, and zoonotic infections are of concern.

[a] Department of Pathobiology, Ontario Veterinary College, University of Guelph, Guelph, Ontario N1G 2W1, Canada; [b] Yu of Guelph Veterinary Dermatology, Guelph Veterinary Specialty Hospital, 1460 Gordon Street South, Guelph, Ontario N1L 1C8, Canada
* Corresponding author.
E-mail address: jsweese@uoguelph.ca

Vet Clin Equine 29 (2013) 559–575
http://dx.doi.org/10.1016/j.cveq.2013.09.004
0749-0739/13/$ – see front matter © 2013 Elsevier Inc. All rights reserved.

Etiology

The *Staphylococcus* genus consists of a large number of different species, including minimally virulent commensals and important opportunistic pathogens. Staphylococci can be differentiated into coagulase-positive and coagulase-negative species (**Table 1**). Coagulase-positive species are the most important clinically, with *Staphylococcus aureus* being the most common cause of staphylococcal disease in horses.[1] However, although it is the most important staphylococcal pathogen it can be found on the skin, mucous membranes, or gastrointestinal tract of a small percentage of healthy horses. The canine-adapted *Staphylococcus pseudintermedius* is the leading cause of bacterial folliculitis in dogs and can also cause disease in horses,[2–4] although this appears to be rare. There is some concern that *S pseudintermedius* may be an emerging pathogen in horses or that it might be misidentified as *S aureus* by diagnostic laboratories, but it is probably an uncommon cause of infection.

Staphylococcus hyicus, a coagulase-variable species, is most often associated with exudative dermatitis in pigs (greasy pig disease), but has been implicated in pastern dermatitis in horses.[5,6] Experimental infection of horses can produce exudative skin lesions,[6] so this species should be considered potentially pathogenic. However, it is an uncommon cause of disease in horses.

Numerous different coagulase-negative staphylococci (CoNS) can be found in or on horses (see **Table 1**), and most healthy horses harbor multiple different CoNS species. Typically, CoNS are of limited virulence and predominantly cause infections in compromised hosts, but infections can occur in immunocompetent animals. Because of the commonness of CoNS in healthy horses and their limited virulence, there may be difficulty differentiating infection from contamination or colonization.

In the past 10 to 15 years, emergence of methicillin-resistant staphylococci has been identified in horses, a factor that has been accompanied by both animal and human health concerns. Methicillin-resistant staphylococci are resistant to virtually all β-lactam antimicrobials (penicillins, cephalosporins, carbapenems) by virtue of the *mecA* gene, and they often have acquired resistance to various other antimicrobial classes. These pathogens can therefore be difficult to treat and are refractory to most drugs used for empiric therapy in horses. Methicillin-resistant *S aureus* (MRSA) has received the most attention in horses because of its ability to cause infections,[7–12]

Table 1
Examples of coagulase-positive and coagulase-negative staphylococci that can be found in horses

Coagulase Positive	Coagulase Negative
S aureus	S epidermidis
S pseudintermedius	S haemolyticus
S delphini	S warneri
S hyicus[a]	S xylosus
	S equorum
	S sciuri
	S felis
	S simulans
	S chromogenes
	S cohnii
	S capitis

[a] Can be coagulase positive or negative.
Data from Refs.[6,49–52]

along with the potential transmission of MRSA between horses and humans,[12–16] and because it appears that MRSA is endemic in the horse population in many regions.[13,16–19] As with methicillin-susceptible *S aureus*, MRSA can be carried by healthy horses,[16,17,20–22] with colonization being much more common than clinical infection. It is apparent that a few major MRSA clones are established in the horse population internationally. One is sequence type 8 (ST8), particularly a strain called USA500 and Canadian epidemic MRSA-5 (CMRSA-5). This human epidemic clone has been found in horses in North America and Europe, and appears to have established itself as an endemic strain in some regions.[12,13,16,19] Recently, the livestock-associated ST398 MRSA has been identified in healthy and diseased horses predominantly in Europe.[13,17,22,23] Other strains, particularly human epidemic clones, have also been found less commonly.

Pathophysiology

Staphylococci are opportunistic pathogens, and primary staphylococcal skin disease occurs rarely (if ever). Factors that affect the body's normal immunologic or physical defenses are critical predisposing factors. Accordingly, wounds, surgical incisions, inflammatory skin conditions, immunosuppressive disorders (eg, Cushing's disease), and skin damage from tack, trauma, or excessive moisture are presumed to be important risk factors for staphylococcal infections. Risk factors for staphylococcal folliculitis, however, have been poorly explored in horses.

Clinical Signs

Staphylococcal folliculitis can present in a variety of ways, ranging from very mild focal and relatively innocuous lesions to rapidly progressive, extensive, and painful disease. Initially, small (1–2 mm) lesions are present, with progression from papules to pustules. These lesions may not be noted initially but can rapidly enlarge and coalesce. Crusts may be present, often in a circular pattern that may lead to empiric (and unsuccessful) ringworm treatment. Epidermal collarettes or encrusted pustules may also be noted.

Pruritus is variable but is usually present, and may be severe. Self-trauma from pruritus may be present and can potentially obscure the underlying staphylococcal lesions. In some cases the affected areas are very painful and edematous, something that is strongly suggestive of staphylococcal dermatitis rather than dermatophilosis or dermatophytosis.

Methicillin resistance does not alter the clinical presentation or progression of disease. These strains are no more inherently virulent than their susceptible counterparts, but more severe disease can occur as a result of failure of empiric treatment.

Diagnosis

Achieving a definitive diagnosis is important because of differences in treatment and overall management of staphylococcal dermatitis in comparison with skin diseases that may have a similar appearance (eg, dermatophilosis, dermatophytosis, *Corynebacterium pseudotuberculosis*). Increasing resistance to commonly used antimicrobials also highlights the need for prompt culture and susceptibility testing. Further, the emergence of MRSA emphasizes the need for additional public health and infection control considerations that are best addressed as early as possible.

Careful clinical examination is required to characterize the disease and to identify optimal areas for sample collection. Small lesions may be overlooked if careful examination is not performed, especially is self-trauma has occurred. Collection of an appropriate diagnostic specimen is critical. Such collection is not always simple, depending on the type and chronicity of lesions, and it is important to maximize the likelihood of recovering the offending organism rather than other bacterial commensals or contaminants. Ideally, samples are collected from intact pustules by opening the pustule with a sterile needle and depositing the material onto a culture swab. Swabs of the undersides of crusts can also be collected but are less preferable. Swabs of the outer surface of older lesions are of little diagnostic utility.

Cytologic examination of the specimen is useful, and often overlooked. Abundant neutrophils with intracellular and extracellular cocci should be present (**Fig. 1**). Bacterial culture and susceptibility testing is a key component of diagnosis and is crucial in guiding therapy. Culture and susceptibility testing should be performed if a good specimen can be obtained. These tests are particularly important when there is severe or rapidly progressive disease, when disease is recurrent, and if initial treatment has failed. Culture results should always be scrutinized carefully. Isolation of coagulase-negative staphylococci should be interpreted with care. Though potentially pathogenic, coagulase-negative staphylococci, including methicillin-resistant strains, are commonly found on healthy skin[24] and are common contaminants. Isolation of a CoNS along with another more convincing pathogen (eg, coagulase-positive *Staphylococcus, Dermatophilus*) should typically be interpreted as contamination. If a CoNS is the only bacterium identified, the diagnosis should be reconsidered, with treatment of the CoNS most justified when there is cytologic evidence of staphylococcal disease and there is no indication that other causes are involved.

Skin biopsies can provide useful information and are particularly important in severe, atypical, nonresponsive, or refractory cases. Multiple biopsies should be collected from areas with active (and ideally new) lesions. Biopsy samples should be submitted for histologic examination and culture.

One aspect of diagnosis that is often overlooked is determination of the underlying cause. Staphylococcal folliculitis is almost always a secondary problem, and efforts to identify health or management factors that predispose to infection are critical. This approach may involve combinations of diagnostic testing (eg, for Cushing's disease, allergies), environmental assessment (eg, stall, turnout areas), and evaluation of management (eg, blanketing, tack, uses that might result in skin trauma, bathing practices).

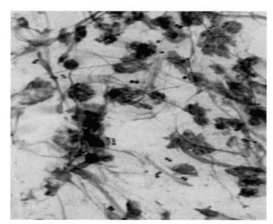

Fig. 1. Cytologic examination of the specimen is useful, and often overlooked. Abundant neutrophils with intracellular and extracellular cocci should be present.

Treatment

Scabs should be removed and the affected area scrubbed with a biocidal soap (eg, 2%–4% chlorhexidine). A contact time of 15 to 30 minutes should be provided before rinsing. Topical therapy is ideally performed daily for the first few days, with less frequent treatment as lesions start to resolve. Sedation may be required if lesions are painful. Analgesic therapy, typically with nonsteroidal anti-inflammatories, may also be required for patient comfort and to reduce self-trauma. Affected areas should be clipped to facilitate cleaning and topical therapy, and to help keep the area dry. Cold hydrotherapy may be beneficial in removing debris, reducing inflammation, and reducing edema. Topical application of antimicrobials such as mupirocin, fusidic acid, or silver sulfadiazine may also be useful with focal superficial infections. Care should be taken to ensure that the horse cannot ingest any topical antimicrobials because of the potential for antimicrobial-associated colitis. Local therapy may be adequate for superficial lesions that are not extensive. Systemic therapy is often required, and treatment should be based on susceptibility-testing results. Penicillin (20,000 IU/kg every 12 hours intramuscularly) may be effective, but the prevalence of β-lactamase production by staphylococci is high. Ceftiofur (ceftiofur sodium 2.2 mg/kg intravenously or intramuscularly every 12 hours, or ceftiofur crystalline free acid 6.6 mg/kg intramuscularly every 4 days) should be effective in the absence of methicillin resistance. Trimethoprim-sulfonamide (24–30 mg/kg by mouth every 12 hours) is often effective, but resistance may be present. There are typically a few viable options for MRSA and other methicillin-resistant staphylococci, but treatment must be guided by susceptibility results because of the potential for resistance to virtually any commonly used drug class.

Treatment should continue until 7 days beyond full clinical resolution. The frequency of adjunctive measures such as hydrotherapy can decrease over time as lesions and associated inflammation improve.

An additional aspect of treatment that cannot be overemphasized is attempting to address any identified or suspected underlying problems through medical, environmental, or management measures. Failure to address underlying risk factors may decrease the likelihood of successful treatment and increase the chance of recurrence.

Prevention

A critical aspect of prevention is reducing the incidence and severity of predisposing factors. In some cases, this may be simple while in others, impossible. Elimination of staphylococci from skin or mucosal reservoirs is not a viable (or desirable) approach. Staphylococci are important components of the commensal skin microbiota, and there is no indication that elimination of staphylococci from skin or mucosal surfaces is either possible or useful. However, there may be instances whereby periodic bathing in biocidal shampoo (eg, 2%–4% chlorhexidine) may be useful to reduce the staphylococcal skin burden on an animal with a flare-up of an underlying condition that might predispose to staphylococcal folliculitis. Prophylactic administration of antimicrobials is not recommended because there is no evidence of efficacy, and it might possibly be associated with increased likelihood of subsequent antimicrobial-resistant infection.

Public Health

Little information is available about risks posed by horses with folliculitis. It is reasonable to assume that there is some risk of zoonotic transmission from contact with infected skin sites, as well as clinically normal skin sites and mucosal surfaces such as nasal passages where staphylococci may reside. *S aureus* is the main public health concern, mainly directed at MRSA. However, if MRSA can be transmitted between horses and humans, it is reasonable to assume that methicillin-susceptible *S aureus* can do the same. Yet the focus of attention is on MRSA because of the significant concerns about this pathogen in human medicine and the clear evidence of transmission of MRSA between horses and humans (in both directions). Zoonotic MRSA infections associated with horses have been reported,[12,14,15] and high rates of MRSA carriage have been identified in people who have contact with horses.[25,26]

Zoonotic risks of other staphylococci, including methicillin-resistant species, are limited. A very small number of methicillin-resistant *S pseudintermedius* (MRSP) infections have been reported in humans[27] and none from horses, but considering the high prevalence of this bacterium in dogs and the low apparent incidence of disease in humans, the risk posed by infected horses is probably limited. Nevertheless, the highly drug-resistant nature of most MRSP strains and the few reported human cases indicate that some degree of prudence is warranted. Close attention to basic hygiene practices is the most important measure.

Infection Control

Because staphylococci are common commensals, isolation of most horses with staphylococcal infections is unnecessary. Some basic infection control and management practices are indicated in routine cases, particularly good hygiene practices (especially hand hygiene), avoidance of contaminating common-use items, preventing the sharing of high-risk items such as blankets, wraps, and brushes, and other measures that would help reduce the risk of direct and indirect transmission of staphylococci. Staphylococci can survive in some environments for weeks, given the appropriate conditions, but they are killed by routine disinfection if done properly. Staphylococci are susceptible to most disinfectants, but the efficacy of disinfectants is often hampered by the surface material (eg, porous surfaces) and organic debris (eg, dirt, pus). Some disinfectants (eg, accelerated hydrogen peroxide) are more effective in contaminated environments, have shorter required contact times, and are compatible with most surfaces. Tack and other items that have been in contact with an infected horse should be laundered and hot-air dried, cleaned and disinfected, or discarded, depending on the surface type and value.

Measures to control MRSA on farms and in equine hospitals are poorly described, but general recommendations can be made based on information from human medicine and basic concepts of infection control and staphylococcal biology (**Box 1**).

DERMATOPHILOSIS
Introduction

Dermatophilosis, also referred to as rain scald or rain rot, is a relatively common exudative and crusting dermatitis in horses. Disease is usually sporadic, although multiple cases can occur on a farm, most likely because of common risk factors (eg, poor stable and turnout management).

Etiology

Dermatophilus congolensis is the etiologic agent. This facultatively anaerobic non–acid-fast gram-positive actinomycete can be found worldwide, particularly in tropical regions, and can infect a wide range of animal species. The bacterium has an unusual life cycle involving 2 forms, hyphae and zoospores. Zoospores are created from

> **Box 1**
> **Measures for the control of methicillin-resistant *Staphylococcus aureus* on farms**
>
> Individual Horse Measures
>
> Isolate infected horses if possible
>
> Use dedicated water buckets, feed bowls, brushes, and other items for affected horses. Decontaminate before using on other horses or discard after use
>
> Use personal protective equipment (dedicated outerwear such as coveralls and gloves) when handling infected horses or entering their stall
>
> Wash hands or use an alcohol-based hand sanitizer after contact with the horse or its environment, including after glove removal
>
> Clean and disinfect the stall after resolution of disease
>
> Turnout only in a dedicated pasture or paddock
>
> Group Measures
>
> Limit antimicrobial use
>
> Cohort horses into different risk groups and limit cross-contact (direct and indirect) between groups
>
> Have a good facility infection control program and preventive medicine program to reduce the risk of opportunistic infections
>
> Quarantine new arrivals
>
> Ensure that culture and susceptibility testing is performed on horses that develop opportunistic infections
>
> Ensure good general hygiene practices by farm personnel and other individuals that have contact with horses (eg, farriers, veterinarians)

coccoid cells that break off the filamentous hyphae, and these represent the infectious stage. Among domestic animals, infections are most often identified in horses, sheep, goats, and cattle, but this bacterium can cause disease in various wild and domestic species.

Epidemiology and Pathophysiology

Dermatophilus congolensis is an opportunist that causes disease secondary to factors that affect the skin integrity and/or immune response (eg, allergies, Cushing's disease, malnutrition). Skin damage (eg, a portal of infection) and/or alteration of the normal skin environment and/or immune system are required for disease to develop following exposure. Despite the commonness of this disease in horses, little research has been published regarding risk factors. However, it is apparent that skin damage from excessive moisture or insect bites and conditions that affect the immune system are the main predisposing causes. Cushing's disease is a particular concern because it can combine an excessive hair coat, increased sweating and moisture trapping, and decreased immune response.

There is limited information about the epidemiology of *D congolensis*, including the prevalence on healthy horses and main routes of transmission. The natural reservoir of this bacterium is unknown, but there may be a wide range of animal hosts. The bacterium can be found on the skin of healthy horses in the absence of disease, and carriers might be an important reservoir. However, the relative role of carriers and diseased horses in transmission is unclear. The bacterium can be transmitted by direct and indirect (eg, fomites) contact. Crusts from infected horses pose the highest risk because of the large bacterial burden. Though perhaps relevant for short-term transmission on farms, the environment probably plays a minimal role in the broader epidemiology.

Clinical Signs

As with most exudative skin diseases, dermatophilosis starts with a papular stage and progresses to pustules. These early abnormalities are often not detected, and disease is not noted until the classic presentation with the development of epidermal collarettes, focal alopecia, coalescing of exudative lesions with matted hair ("paint-brush lesions") and thick crusts. Crusts are easily removable, with abundant pus underneath and potential bleeding caused by skin erosion (**Fig. 2**A).[28] As disease progresses, there is typically less purulent discharge and dry crusts may predominate. Pruritus is variable. Lesions may be regional or generalized, with lesion distribution being representative of the underlying cause, such as areas where excessive moisture is present (ie, dorsum, race, rump), where biting insects prefer, or where skin trauma is common (ie, girth and saddle area, lower limbs). Crust and scab formation is most common with longer hair coats, so in temperate climates the appearance of lesions in summer differs from that in winter.

Diagnosis

Clinical appearance is strongly suggestive, particularly in horses that are kept in wet environments or with other recognized risk factors. Impression smears of the undersides of crusts are very useful because of the characteristic "railroad-track" cytologic appearance of the bacterium (see **Fig. 2**B). Early lesions with ample exudate are optimal. Crusts can be plucked and pressed onto a glass slide. Alternatively, crusts can be mixed with saline and macerated before placing on a slide, a technique that is most effective for older or dry lesions.

Definitive diagnosis is based on isolation of the bacterium from crusts or biopsies, although this is uncommonly performed as an initial diagnostic test. Alternatively, histopathology may be used for diagnosis. A thick crust composed of palisading layers of parakeratotic stratum corneum, dried serum, and degenerating neutrophils is the most characteristic change (see **Fig. 2**C). A superficial folliculitis may be a prominent feature

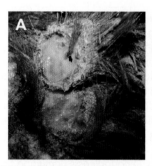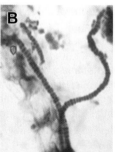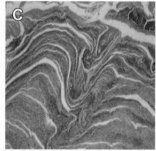

Fig. 2. (A) Thick crust with purulent exudate peeled off the skin from a patient with dermatophilosis. (B) Cytologic appearance of *Dermatophilus congolensis*. Note the filamentous appearance of chains of parallel "railroad-track" gram-positive cocci. (C) Thick crust from a patient with dermatophilosis, composed of palisading layers of parakeratotic stratum corneum, dried serum, and degenerating neutrophils, which constitute the most characteristic change. Organisms are typically sandwiched between the layers.

of the disease. In sections stained with Gram stain, the branching, filamentous organisms can be observed in the crusts and in the follicles. More extensive diagnostic testing should be considered to rule out other conditions or concurrent infections, particularly in atypical cases or those that fail to respond as expected.

Consideration of the underlying problem should also be part of the diagnostic process. This approach can involve investigation of environmental factors and management, or diagnostic testing (eg, diagnosis of Cushing's disease, intradermal allergy testing).

Treatment

Infection can be self-limiting if underlying problems are corrected, but specific therapy is usually indicated. Affected horses should be kept in a dry environment to facilitate skin healing. Crusts should be gently removed after soaking with biocidal shampoo or rinses (eg, 2%–4% chlorhexidine, benzoyl peroxide). Vigorous scrubbing should be avoided. Clipping affected areas and adjacent areas can facilitate topical therapy and maintain a dry skin environment. Antibacterial shampoos or rinses containing 2% to 4% chlorhexidine, benzoyl peroxide, accelerated hydrogen peroxide, or other nonirritating biocides should be used. A 10- to 15-minute contact time should be provided before rinsing.[28] Bathing should occur every 1 to 2 days initially, and at least once weekly until 1 week after clinical resolution. Focal lesions can be treated more often with biocidal sprays or ointments (eg, 4% chlorhexidine spray). Topical antimicrobials such as mupirocin or fusidic acid should also be effective, but it is unclear whether they confer much more benefit than topical biocides.

Systemic antimicrobials can be considered, but are rarely needed. It is ideal to reserve systemic antimicrobials for severe or refractory cases or for cases whereby topical therapy is not possible. Systemic therapy can be effective, but is accompanied by a risk of antimicrobial-associated complications (eg, diarrhea) and emergence of antimicrobial resistant pathogens. If systemic therapy is elected, bathing and removal of crusts should be performed if possible. D congolensis is almost always susceptible to a wide range of antimicrobials, with penicillin (20,000 IU/kg intramuscularly every 12 hours until 1 week after clinical resolution of lesion) being the drug of choice.

Concurrent measures to address any identified underlying problems are critical. This approach may involve changes in housing (eg, providing better cover outside, improving ventilation), management (eg, blanketing practices, improved nutrition), ectoparasite control, or treatment of underlying diseases (eg, allergies, Cushing's disease).

Prevention

Prevention involves good management and animal care practices that reduce predisposing causes, particularly ensuring that horses have access to proper shelter, and control of biting flies.

Public Health

Human infections have been reported, but are rare and mainly occur in tropical regions.[29] Although the potential for zoonotic transmission should not be dismissed, considering the incidence of this disease in horses, the limited use of strict infection control and hygiene measures around infected horses, and the paucity of reports of human infection (especially infections linked to horses), the risk is exceedingly low. Basic hygiene practices, particularly good attention to hand hygiene after handling infected horses, wearing some form of protective outerwear (eg, coveralls) when bathing infected horses, and other basic barrier protection approaches, should be adequate. People with skin lesions or underlying skin disease should be particularly careful and use rigorous hand-hygiene practices. Alcohol-based hand sanitizers should be highly effective against this bacterium, and equally as effective as hand washing.

Infection Control

Multiple cases of dermatophilosis can occur in the same group of horses, although this relates largely to commonness of the underlying problem. Presumably this bacterium can be exchanged readily through direct or indirect (eg, fomites) means, and basic practices can reduce any risks. Crusts may pose the greatest risk, so care must be taken not to contaminate the environment or items during crust removal and patient treatment. Tack, blankets, and other items that have contact with the skin should not be shared between infected and uninfected horses. Items used on infected horses should be cleaned and disinfected after resolution of infection and/or before use on another horse. Many items are difficult to thoroughly disinfect, but the limited risk of transmission decreases concern about low-level residual bacterial contamination. Blankets, wraps, and similar items should be washed and hot-air dried. Items that cannot be laundered should be cleaned and ideally be sprayed with a routine disinfectant; however, surface compatibility must be considered. Routine cleaning and disinfection of the stall should be adequate. Infected horses do not require strict isolation; rather, keeping them away from other horses during the early treatment period, when bacterial burdens are highest, is a prudent measure. Particular care should be taken to avoid direct or indirect contact with horses that have underlying skin disease or immunosuppressive disorders (eg, Cushing's disease). A single case report of *D congolensis* placentitis and abortion in a mare exists,[30] so it may be prudent to adopt a stricter approach around pregnant mares, although the risk is presumably low.

Personnel working with an infected horse should use contact precautions to reduce the risk of transmission to other horses, low as it may be.

DERMATOPHYTOSIS

Dermatophytosis, commonly referred to as ringworm, is an important and highly contagious fungal infection caused by dermatophytes of the *Microsporum* and *Trichophyton* genera. Though of limited morbidity, ringworm can be problematic because of the potential for outbreaks, prolonged disease (at the individual or herd levels), cost and bother of treatment, and the potential for human infection.

Etiology

Dermatophytes are keratinophilic fungi. A wide range of dermatophyte species exist, which can be divided into zoophilic and geophilic groups. Most animal infections are caused by zoophilic species, with *Trichophyton equinum* and *Microsporum canis* (also referred to as *Microsporum equinum*) most common in horses,[31-33] and *T equinum* predominating in older horses.[32] Other species such as *Trichophyton mentagrophytes*, *Trichophyton verrucosum*, and *Trichophyton bullosum*, and the geophilic *Microsporum gypseum,* may be found occasionally in some regions.[32,34]

Epidemiology and Pathophysiology

The incidence of disease and prevalence of dermatophyte shedding are poorly characterized in horses. Dermatophytes can be found on a small percentage of healthy horses,[31] but it is unclear whether equine infections originate mainly from clinically infected horses or clinically normal equine carriers. Horses can also be infected by other animal species, such as dogs, cats, and cattle, although the importance of these sources is unknown.

Zoophilic dermatophytes are transmitted by direct contact with infected animals or contact with arthroconidia (spores) in the environment or on fomites (eg, tack, blankets). Specific risk factors for horses have not been adequately investigated, although one study reported a higher incidence of disease on training farms than on breeding farms.[35] A study of Australian thoroughbreds identified a predominance of lesions in the girth area, supporting tack as an important route of transmission.[36] Young age (<3 years) and high humidity were also risk factors. Geophilic species are found in the environment, and contact with contaminated environments, particularly soil, is the main source of exposure.

Dermatophytes have keratinophilic and keratinolytic properties,[32] and clinical infection involves the superficial keratinized layers of the hair coat and skin.[37] After exposure, dermatophyte arthroconidia attach and germinate, then invade the stratum corneum, a process that takes approximately 3 days in human explant models[38]; and a similar time frame is likely present in horses. Clinical disease is usually apparent within 9 to 15 days of exposure.[39] Protease production digests keratin, providing a nutritional source and initiating skin and hair damage.[37] Differences in keratinase production can be present between strains, which may account for apparent differences in clinical virulence. Other factors also contribute to host damage, including the host immune response, host protease secretion, and various other likely pathogen and host factors.[37] An effective delayed-type hypersensitivity cell-mediated immune response is required for elimination of infection.[37] Animals with compromised immune systems may therefore develop more serious or more prolonged disease.

The reason why dermatophytes can be found on the skin and hair coat of animals without disease is unclear. It is possible that low-level exposure and an effective immune response result in temporary colonization with no disease, but this has not been adequately studied.

Clinical Signs

Classically, a circular area of alopecia and scaling with an erythematous margin is evident.[32] Lesions may grow centripetally, and with time there may be resolution of infection in central areas with new hair growth while active disease continues to extend outward (**Fig. 3**). However, this classic presentation is not always present, and affected animals can have variable distributions and shapes of affected areas. There may be single lesions or multiple lesions in a cluster or widely disseminated. The head, neck, and forelimbs are most commonly affected. Spread over the body may be rapid, particularly in young animals. Pruritus is uncommon but may be present in some animals. Close examination of affected areas may reveal papules and pustules,[28] depending on the age of the lesion. The classic appearance is not always present in horses, and in some cases the main signs are less pronounced, with broken hairs, small alopecic areas, and a hair coat that looks more "rough" than diseased.

Diagnosis

Consideration of dermatophytosis is important for any horse with dermatologic disease because of the variable clinical presentation and potential for rapid spread. Clinical appearance can provide a suspicion of ringworm, but confirmation should take place to rule out other similar-appearing conditions (eg, dermatophilosis, staphylococcal folliculitis) and atypical presentations of ringworm.

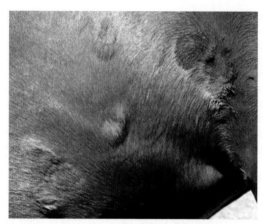

Fig. 3. Common dermatophytic lesions consist of a circular area of alopecia and scaling, with centripetal spreading and resolution of infection in central areas with new hair growth, while active disease continues to extend outward.

Wood's lamp can be used as a screening tool; however, false negatives are common because not all dermatophytes fluoresce. Negative results should never be used to rule out dermatophytosis. Wood's lamp is most effective as a monitoring tool when a fluorescing strain of *M canis (M equinum)* is known to be present in a group or on an individual. Fluorescence is best observed during early or active infection, when the entire hair shaft will fluoresce,[32] as later in disease only the most distal components will fluoresce. Wood's lamp can be useful for selection of optimal sites to collect samples for fungal culture.

Direct microscopic examination of infected hairs (trichoscopy) collected by plucking or skin scraping has provided variable success. After digestion with 10% to 20% potassium hydroxide to remove keratin and associated debris, dermatophytes can be noted in clusters or chains along the hair surface (**Fig. 4**).[32,40] Direct staining with Giemsa stain may also be used to visualize arthroconidia, although this is likely of lower sensitivity.

Adhesive tape impression (ATI) is used to collect and secure hair samples of affected and unaffected hairs, which are then placed onto a glass slide for microscopic evaluation. The sample is examined either directly using low-power (4×–10× objective) for evidence of ectothrix. Packing tape (such as 3M ScotchPad Packaging

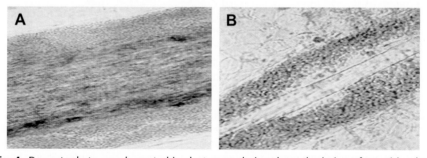

Fig. 4. Dermatophytes can be noted in clusters or chains along the hair surface with a lactophenol cotton blue stain used to enhance the spore along the hair shaft. (*A*) *Microsporum canis*. (*B*) *Microsporum gypseum*.

Tape Pad 3750PY) is used in preference to regular clear Scotch tape, as the former is stickier (especially useful for collecting affected hairs) and tends not to curl as readily when adhering to a slide. ATI is the sampling method of choice for dermatophyte evaluation, as it adheres fragile infected hairs rather than leaving the broken infected hairs behind when sampling with hemostats.

Fungal culture is the gold standard. Hair should be collected from clinically affected areas, with new lesions preferred. Hair is collected by plucking or toothbrush sampling. Biopsies can also be cultured, as can debris from skin scrapings. A diagnostic laboratory that has experience with dermatophyte isolation and identification is preferred. Selective media are required to prevent overgrowth of various environmental and commensal fungi. Commercial in-clinic assays are available. These assays can allow for a preliminary diagnosis based on colony morphology and color change of medium, but suspected positive cases should always be confirmed via microscopy or submission to a diagnostic laboratory to prevent false-positive diagnoses. An additional consideration is the biosafety requirements for in-clinic culture. Containment at biosafety level 2 should be used to reduce the risk of laboratory-associated infection. These practices are feasible in a veterinary clinic, but require consideration of physical layout, training, cleaning and disinfection, decontamination, and waste disposal.

Treatment

Ringworm is a self-limiting disease in immunocompetent animals,[32] although 1 to 4 months may be required.[41] Treatment typically is pursued to hasten recovery and reduce the risk of subsequent human or animal infections.

Topical and systemic options are available, and little objective information is available regarding optimal approaches in horses. Topical therapy can be effective alone or in conjunction with systemic treatment, and should be considered for all cases.[28] Affected areas can be clipped to facilitate treatment. Clippers and clipper blades should be disinfected after use. Scabs should be removed and disposed of in a manner that will not contaminate the environment. All lesions and the surrounding hair coat should be treated. Ideally the entire hair coat is treated because dermatophytes may be present widely over the body, not just at visibly affected sites. A wide range of topical options are available in rinse or shampoo formulations, including enilconazole 0.2% (Imaverol), natamycin, ketoconazole 1% to 2%, miconazole, chlorhexidine 2% to 4%, and combinations of ketoconazole and chlorhexidine.[28,42] A 2% lime sulfur solution is effective but is undesirable because of the odor and potential for staining of light hair coats.[32] Accelerated hydrogen peroxide may be another topical treatment option because of its efficacy against dermatophytes, but data are currently limited. Terbinafine 1% or miconazole 2% can be used as spot treatments but are not practical for treatment of the whole animal. Natamycin suspension is also useful for focal topical therapy.[41] Treatment intervals are not well described, and range from daily to weekly. At least 2 to 3 treatments per week should be administered initially.

Limited information is available about the safety and efficacy of systemic antifungals. Griseofulvin (5–10 mg/kg or 100 mg/kg by mouth every 24 hours) is occasionally used, although evidence of superiority to topical therapy is lacking. The variable reported dosing ranges question the efficacy of this product in equine dermatology. Griseofulvin is a teratogen, and should not be used in pregnant mares. Whereas medications such as itraconazole and fluconazole have been used to treat horses with systemic mycotic infections such as coccidioidomycosis and aspergillosis, there have not been any studies on their effectiveness in dermatophytosis. However, their safety record in horses in the face of the doses used (2–5 mg/kg every 12 hours) is encouraging.[43–45] Terbinafine is widely used in dogs and cats, and although pharmacokinetics of this drug have been investigated in horses,[46] efficacy data are limited to a weak uncontrolled study of 2 horses that reported clinical cure (albeit for a typically self-limiting disease).[47] Alternatively, sodium iodide 20% may be given intravenously (250 mL/500 kg horse every 7 days, 1 to 2 times), although this also is contraindicated in pregnant mares as it may cause abortion.

Considering the cost and potential toxicity of oral antifungal medication, combined with the self-limiting nature of disease and relative ease of topical therapy, topical therapy alone is a reasonable approach, with oral treatment reserved for refractory or perhaps severe cases. Oral treatment is best reserved for situations whereby topical therapy cannot be performed adequately because of the horse's temperament or inability to bathe because of cold weather. Treatment typically is continued for 2 to 4 weeks after resolution of clinical signs, and after 2 negative cultures (collected 3–7 days apart) have been obtained.[41]

Prevention

There are no specific preventive measures. Vaccination has been shown to provide a reasonable degree of protection in horses,[48] but equine vaccines are not commercially available in most regions. General infection-control practices, including quarantine of new arrivals, preventing sharing of tack and other skin-contact items, and prompt diagnosis of suspected cases, are important, in addition to specific measures used in response to suspected or confirmed cases (see later discussion). Prophylactic topical treatment of exposed horses can be considered. If used tack is purchased, it should be cleaned and disinfected before use. Used blankets should be laundered and hot-air dried.

Public Health

Dermatophytosis is a common zoonotic disease, although horses are uncommonly implicated in human infections. The risk varies between different dermatophytes, with *M canis* posing the greatest risk.[32] Any infected horse poses a risk to humans through direct contact or through contact with contaminated fomites. The incidence of zoonotic ringworm in people in contact with infected horses is unknown, although all infected horses should be considered infectious.

Infection Control

Infected horses should be isolated to prevent direct or indirect contact with other horses and to facilitate the use of proper infection-control practices. Dermatophytes are spread through contact, not aerosol or airborne routes, so isolation within a main barn is acceptable as long as there is no potential for horse-horse contact around doors or over walls. If the potential for contact exists, temporary barriers should be erected or empty stalls should be left on either side. If infected horses are turned out, an individual pasture or paddock should be used, and there should be no potential for contact with other horses over fences. If affected horses are walked, personnel should be diligent to ensure there is no transient contact with other horses.

Dermatophytes can survive for months to years in the environment and on tack under the appropriate conditions.[32,36] Therefore, potentially contaminated areas and items should be cleaned and disinfected, and this should be done periodically during the treatment period. A thorough terminal cleaning and disinfection should be performed after resolution of infection. Disinfection of stalls may be difficult if unsealed wood, concrete, or dirt surfaces are present, but removal of as much organic debris as possible, thorough washing, and application of a disinfectant with antidermatophyte activity (eg, accelerated hydrogen peroxide, 1:10 concentration of household bleach) should markedly reduce any dermatophyte burden and subsequent risk.

Items that have come into contact with infected horses should also be considered infectious. Items such as buckets and brushes should be soaked in disinfectant and thoroughly rinsed after 15 minutes' contact time. Blankets, wraps, and other items that can be laundered should be laundered and hot-air dried. Disinfection of tack can difficult because many items have porous surfaces. Tack should be thoroughly washed and sprayed with a disinfectant. Accelerated hydrogen peroxide is probably less damaging than bleach to surfaces, and is preferred. After 15 minutes' contact time, tack should be rinsed to remove residual disinfectant.

Contact with infected horses should be minimized. Personal protective equipment should be worn whenever horses are handled or when the stall is entered. The most important components are an item that covers the clothing (eg, coveralls) and is only used for the infected horse, and gloves. Protective outerwear should be stored so that it does not cross-contaminate other items, and should be donned and removed with care to avoid inadvertent contamination of the hands or other parts of the body. Hands must be washed after removal of gloves.

REFERENCES

1. Panchaud Y, Gerber V, Rossano A, et al. Bacterial infections in horses: a retrospective study at the University Equine Clinic of Bern. Schweiz Arch Tierheilkd 2010;152:176–82.
2. De Martino L, Lucido M, Mallardo K, et al. Methicillin-resistant staphylococci isolated from healthy horses and horse personnel in Italy. J Vet Diagn Invest 2010; 22:77–82.
3. Haenni M, Targant H, Forest K, et al. Retrospective study of necropsy-associated coagulase-positive staphylococci in horses. J Vet Diagn Invest 2010;22:953–6.
4. Devriese L, Hermans K, Baele M, et al. Staphylococcus pseudintermedius versus Staphylococcus intermedius. Vet Microbiol 2009;133:206–7.
5. Devriese LA, Nzuambe D, Godard C. Identification and characteristics of staphylococci isolated from lesions and normal skin of horses. Vet Microbiol 1985;10: 269–77.
6. Devriese LA, Vlaminck K, Nuytten J, et al. Staphylococcus hyicus in skin lesions of horses. Equine Vet J 1983;15:263–5.
7. Anderson ME, Lefebvre SL, Rankin SC, et al. Retrospective multicentre study of methicillin-resistant Staphylococcus aureus infections in 115 horses. Equine Vet J 2009;41:401–5.
8. Bergstrom K, Aspan A, Landen A, et al. The first nosocomial outbreak of methicillin-resistant Staphylococcus aureus in horses in Sweden. Acta Vet Scand 2012;54:11.
9. Hartmann FA, Trostle SS, Klohnen AA. Isolation of methicillin-resistant Staphylococcus aureus from a postoperative wound infection in a horse. J Am Vet Med Assoc 1997;211:590–2.
10. Maeda Y, Millar BC, Loughrey A, et al. Community-associated MRSA SCCmec type IVd in Irish equids. Vet Rec 2007;161:35–6.
11. Seguin JC, Walker RD, Caron JP, et al. Methicillin-resistant Staphylococcus aureus outbreak in a veterinary teaching hospital: potential human-to-animal transmission. J Clin Microbiol 1999;37:1459–63.

12. Weese JS, Archambault M, Willey BM, et al. Methicillin-resistant *Staphylococcus aureus* in horses and horse personnel, 2000-2002. Emerg Infect Dis 2005;11: 430–5.
13. van Duijkeren E, Moleman M, Sloet van Oldruitenborgh-Oosterbaan M, et al. Methicillin-resistant *Staphylococcus aureus* in horses and horse personnel: an investigation of several outbreaks. Vet Microbiol 2010;141:96–102.
14. van Duijkeren E, Ten Horn L, Wagenaar JA, et al. Suspected horse-to-human transmission of MRSA ST398. Emerg Infect Dis 2011;17:1137–9.
15. Weese JS, Caldwell F, Willey BM, et al. An outbreak of methicillin-resistant *Staphylococcus aureus* skin infections resulting from horse to human transmission in a veterinary hospital. Vet Microbiol 2005;114:160–4.
16. Weese JS, Rousseau J, Traub-Dargatz JL, et al. Community-associated methicillin-resistant *Staphylococcus aureus* in horses and humans who work with horses. J Am Vet Med Assoc 2005;226:580–3.
17. Van den Eede A, Martens A, Lipinska U, et al. High occurrence of methicillin-resistant *Staphylococcus aureus* ST398 in equine nasal samples. Vet Microbiol 2009;133:138–44.
18. Weese JS, Lefebvre SL. Risk factors for methicillin-resistant *Staphylococcus aureus* colonization in horses admitted to a veterinary teaching hospital. Can Vet J 2007;48:921–6.
19. Weese JS, Rousseau J, Willey BM, et al. Methicillin-resistant *Staphylococcus aureus* in horses at a veterinary teaching hospital: frequency, characterization, and association with clinical disease. J Vet Intern Med 2006;20: 182–6.
20. Maddox TW, Clegg PD, Diggle PJ, et al. Cross-sectional study of antimicrobial-resistant bacteria in horses. Part 1: prevalence of antimicrobial-resistant Escherichia coli and methicillin-resistant Staphylococcus aureus. Equine Vet J 2012; 44(3):289–96.
21. Van den Eede A, Hermans K, Van den Abeele A, et al. Methicillin-resistant *Staphylococcus aureus* (MRSA) on the skin of long-term hospitalised horses. Vet J 2012;193:408–11.
22. Van den Eede A, Martens A, Feryn I, et al. Low MRSA prevalence in horses at farm level. BMC Vet Res 2012;8:213.
23. Tokateloff N, Manning ST, Weese JS, et al. Prevalence of methicillin-resistant *Staphylococcus aureus* colonization in horses in Saskatchewan, Alberta, and British Columbia. Can Vet J 2009;50:1177–80.
24. Vengust M, Anderson ME, Rousseau J, et al. Methicillin-resistant staphylococcal colonization in clinically normal dogs and horses in the community. Lett Appl Microbiol 2006;43:602–6.
25. Anderson ME, Lefebvre SL, Weese JS. Evaluation of prevalence and risk factors for methicillin-resistant *Staphylococcus aureus* colonization in veterinary personnel attending an international equine veterinary conference. Vet Microbiol 2008;129:410–7.
26. Hanselman BA, Kruth SA, Rousseau J, et al. Methicillin-resistant *Staphylococcus aureus* colonization in veterinary personnel. Emerg Infect Dis 2006;12: 1933–8.
27. Stegmann R, Burnens A, Maranta CA, et al. Human infection associated with methicillin-resistant *Staphylococcus pseudintermedius* ST71. J Antimicrob Chemother 2010;65:2047–8.
28. Marsella R. Dermatophilosis. In: Sellon DC, Long MT, editors. Equine infectious diseases. St Louis (MO): Saunders Elsevier; 2007. p. 409–12.

29. Amor A, Enríquez A, Corcuera MT, et al. Is infection by *Dermatophilus congolensis* underdiagnosed? J Clin Microbiol 2011;49:449–51.
30. Sebastian MM, Giles RC, Donahu JM, et al. Dermatophilus congolensis-associated placentitis, funisitis and abortion in a horse. Transbound Emerg Dis 2008;55:183–5.
31. Moretti A, Boncio L, Pasquali P, et al. Epidemiological aspects of dermatophyte infections in horses and cattle. Zentralbl Veterinarmed B 1998;45:205–8.
32. Chermette R, Ferreiro L, Guillot J. Dermatophytoses in animals. Mycopathologia 2008;166:385–405.
33. de Vries GA, Jitta CR. An epizootic in horses in the Netherlands caused by *Trichophyton equinum* var. *equinum*. Sabouraudia 1973;11:137–9.
34. Sitterle E, Frealle E, Foulet F, et al. *Trichophyton bullosum*: a new zoonotic dermatophyte species. Med Mycol 2012;50:305–9.
35. Pascoe RR. Studies on the prevalence of ringworm among horses in racing and breeding stables. Aust Vet J 1976;52:419–21.
36. Pascoe RR. The epidemiology of ringworm in racehorses caused by *Trichophyton equinum* var *autotrophicum*. Aust Vet J 1979;55:403–7.
37. Vermout S, Tabart J, Baldo A, et al. Pathogenesis of dermatophytosis. Mycopathologia 2008;166:267–75.
38. Duek L, Kaufman G, Ulman Y, et al. The pathogenesis of dermatophyte infections in human skin sections. J Infect 2004;48:175–80.
39. Pascoe JR. Skin. In: Munroe GA, Weese JS, editors. Equine clinical medicine, surgery and reproduction. London: Manson Publishing Ltd; 2011. p. 873–938.
40. Robert R, Pihet M. Conventional methods for the diagnosis of dermatophytosis. Mycopathologia 2008;166:295–306.
41. Cafarchia C, Figueredo LA, Otranto D. Fungal diseases of horses. Vet Microbiol 2013;1–20.
42. Oldenkamp EP. Treatment of ringworm in horses with natamycin. Equine Vet J 1979;11:36–8.
43. Foley JP, Legendre AM. Treatment of coccidioidomycosis osteomyelitis with itraconazole in a horse. A brief report. J Vet Intern Med 1992;6:333–4.
44. Korenek NL, Legendre AM, Andrews FM, et al. Treatment of mycotic rhinitis with itraconazole in three horses. J Vet Intern Med 1994;8:224–7.
45. Taintor J, Crowe C, Hancock S, et al. Treatment of conidiobolomycosis with fluconazole in two pregnant mares. J Vet Intern Med 2004;18:363–4.
46. Williams MM, Davis EG, KuKanich B. Pharmacokinetics of oral terbinafine in horses and Greyhound dogs. J Vet Pharmacol Ther 2011;34:232–7.
47. Burkhart CG, Burkhart KM. Dermatophytosis in horses treated with terbinafine. J Equine Vet Sci 1999;19:652–3.
48. Pier AC, Zancanella PJ. Immunization of horses against dermatophytosis caused by *Trichophyton equinum*. Equine Pract 1993;15:23–7.
49. Kern A, Perreten V. Clinical and molecular features of methicillin-resistant, coagulase-negative staphylococci of pets and horses. J Antimicrob Chemother 2013; 68(6):1256–66.
50. Karakulska J, Fijałkowski K, Nawrotek P, et al. Identification and methicillin resistance of coagulase-negative staphylococci isolated from nasal cavity of healthy horses. J Microbiol 2012;50:444–51.
51. Biberstein EL, Jang SS, Hirsh DC. Species distribution of coagulase-positive staphylococci in animals. J Clin Microbiol 1984;19:610–5.
52. Cox HU, Newman SS, Roy AF, et al. Species of Staphylococcus isolated from animal infections. Cornell Vet 1984;74:124–35.

Equine Pastern Dermatitis

Anthony A. Yu, DVM, MS

KEYWORDS

- Pastern dermatitis • Lymphedema • Leukocytoclastic vasculitis • Grease heel
- Scratches

KEY POINTS

- Equine Pastern Dermatitis is a syndrome and not a diagnosis. The identification of primary, perpetuating and predisposing factors is key to determining an appropriate and successful treatment course.
- Pastern Leukocytoclastic vasculitis is an immune-mediated condition that requires glucocorticoids as part of the initial treatment regimen while addressing secondary antimicrobial infections. Pentoxifylline is often used concurrently to aid with microvascular bloodflow and act as a steroid-sparing agent.
- Acetate tape impressions are minimally invasive and can provide diagnostic formation regarding ectoparasites, bacteria, yeast and dermatophytic infections. Use of clear packing tape and Diff Quik stains (omitting the alcohol dip) allows better differentiation of infectious organisms.
- Eprinomectin is a topical parasiticide with known activity of psoroptic mange and anecdotal efficacy against chorioptic mange in horses. As chorioptic mites are surface feeders, eprinomectin may provide better efficacy than systemically administered macrocyclic lactones.

INTRODUCTION

Equine Pastern Dermatitis (EPD) is not a single disease, but a cutaneous reaction pattern of the horse. EPD should be considered a syndrome, rather than a diagnosis.[1,2] Uncovering the underlying etiology prior to treatment is key to minimizing treatment failures and frustration. To achieve a positive therapeutic outcome, treating the predisposing and perpetuating factors isjust as important as addressing the primary cause of EPD (**Fig. 1**).[2]

CLINICAL SIGNS AND PATHOGENESIS

EPD can affect any breed of horses, but it is most commonly seen in draft horses.[1,2] Feathering over the pasterns is a predisposing factor.[1,3] EPD occurs without a sex predilection and is seen mostly in adult horses.[1–4] The dermatitis usually affects the caudal aspect of the pasterns, with the hind limbs most commonly affected.[2,5] If not

Yu of Guelph Veterinary Dermatology, Guelph Veterinary Specialty Hospital, 1460 Gordon Street South, Guelph, Ontario N1L 1C8, Canada
E-mail address: yuvetpc@gmail.com

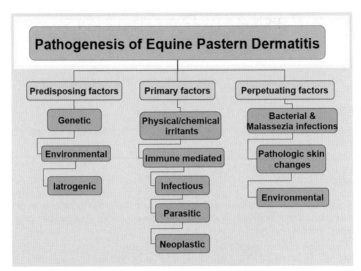

Fig. 1. EPD is a descriptive term and not a diagnosis. The flow chart of depicts the potential primary, predisposing, and perpetuating factors of EPD.

addressed, the lesions can spread anteriorly to involve the front of the pastern and fetlock areas.[1,2] The lesions are bilaterally symmetric; however, they can affect just 1 limb. Lesions are more often detected on, but are not limited to the nonpigmented areas of the pasterns.[5] Clinical signs will vary depending on the etiology, duration, and previous therapy. Initially, there is edema, erythema, and scaling, which rapidly progress to exudation, matting of the hair, and crusting.[1,2,5] If the underlying cause is vasculitis, ulcers may be noted.[2,5] Secondary bacterial infection is a common complication and perpetuating factor.[1,2] With chronicity, the skin may become thickened and fissured because of the constant movement and flexion in this area.[5] The lesions are often painful and can result in lameness.[5]

There are 3 different presentations:

1. Mild form (scratches, mud fever, mud rash). This is the mildest and most prevalent form of EPD. There is alopecia, dry scales, and crusts. The skin can be thickened, and pruritus and pain are variable (**Fig. 2**).

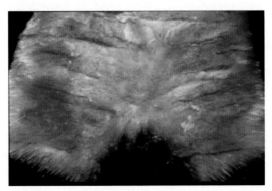

Fig. 2. Mild form (scratches, mud fever, mud rash). This is the mildest and most prevalent form of EPD. There is alopecia, dry scales, and crusts. (*Courtesy of* Valerie Fadok, DVM, PhD, DACVD, North Houston Veterinary Specialists, Texas.)

2. Exudative form (grease heel, dew poisoning). This type is a more exudative form of EPD. One may observe erythema, erosion, alopecia, and serous to purulent crusting dermatitis. Often accompanying epidermolysis and vasculitis are present (**Fig. 3**).

3. Chronic proliferative form (grapes, verrucous pododermatitis).[2,6,7] This form is characterized by excessive granulation tissue (fibroblastic proliferation) that becomes cornified. Nodular proliferations of hyperkeratosis and lichenification can be seen. Fissures and papillomatous areas may develop, and their formation is a common sequela in draft breeds (**Fig. 4**).[2,6,8]

A condition characterized by progressive swelling, hyperkeratosis, and fibrosis of the distal limbs in Shires, Clydesdales, and Belgian Draft horses has been under investigation at the University of California, Davis (UC Davis).[9] The clinical signs and pathologic changes are similar to a condition in people known as chronic lymphedema or elephantiasis. Factors that have been proposed to contribute to this disease are abnormal functioning lymphatic system in the skin, which causes severe swelling and fibrosis, a compromised immune system, and secondary skin infections.[10] The lesions do not respond well to therapy. As the disease progresses and becomes more chronic, the enlarged lower extremity becomes permanent, and the swelling is firm on palpation.[10] There is progressive skin fold and nodule formation that are first noted on the posterior aspect of the pastern. With chronicity, the nodules and folds occupy the entire lower extremity (**Fig. 5**). Over time, the affected limb will result in mobility problems, which is often traumatized during normal exercise. The prognosis is poor due to the development of secondary infections, poor response to therapy, systemic illness, and debilitation. Recently, however, the group at UC Davis studied combined decongestive therapy (CDT), which includes manual lymph drainage (MLD) and subsequent bandaging with short stretch bandages.[11] With CDT, a mean volume reduction of 4.75% to 21.74% was achieved, resulting in increased mobility and purposeful movement. As CDT is not readily available in Canada, the author has used an oral medication combining low-dose dexamethasone along with trichlormethiazide, a diuretic. This combination of medications has been licensed for treatment of udder edema in cattle and is sold as Naquasone in an injectable or bolus form. Formulated into an oral paste, it offers cost-effective palliative therapy for the Chronic Progressive Lymphedema (CPL) equine owner.

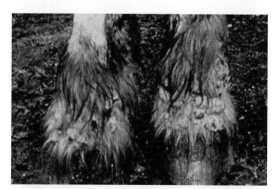

Fig. 3. Exudative form (grease heel, dew poisoning). This type is a more exudative form of EPD. One may observe erythema, erosion, alopecia, and serous to purulent crusting dermatitis. (*Courtesy of* Valerie Fadok, DVM, PhD, DACVD, North Houston Veterinary Specialists, Texas.)

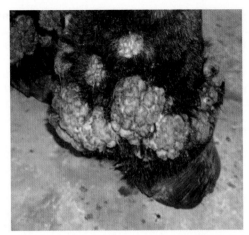

Fig. 4. Chronic proliferative form-(grapes, *Verrucous pododermatitis*). This form is characterized by excessive granulation tissue (fibroblastic proliferation) that becomes cornified. Nodular proliferations of hyperkeratosis and lichenification can be seen. (*Courtesy of* Luc Beco, DVM, DECVD Cabinet Veterinaire Pour Animaux de Compagnie, Avenue Reine Astrid, Belgium.)

Pastern leukocytoclastic vasculitis (PLV) (photo-aggravated vasculitis) is an additional clinical cause of EPD. This disease is poorly understood and affects mature horses. It is unique to the horse and affects primarily unpigmented distal extremities.[5,12] It is believed to be an immune complex disease.[5] If immune complexes are involved in the pathogenesis, their deposition in the distal limbs may be due to regional vasculature differences.[5] Clinical signs suggest it is a photo-aggravated condition and hence is seen mainly in the summer. Lesions are multiple and consist of well-demarcated circular painful, erythematous, exudative, tightly adherent crusts

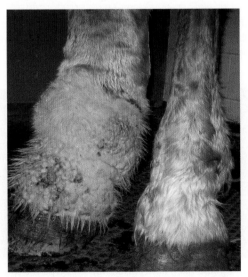

Fig. 5. Chronic progressive lymphedema with progressive skin fold and nodule formation first noted on the posterior aspect of the pastern. With chronicity, the nodules and folds occupy the entire lower extremity.

(**Fig. 6**). Patients often present to orthopedic surgeons with a suspicion of a muscle tear or skeletal injury.[13] The medial and lateral aspects of the pasterns are the areas most commonly affected. Lesions appear painful rather than pruritic. Edema of limb and lameness are common sequelae. Chronic cases may develop a rough or warty surface.[5] Differential diagnoses for dermatitis of the distal limbs that is not restricted to nonpigmented skin include, but are not limited to, primary irritant or allergic contact dermatitis, pastern folliculitis/pyoderma (eg, *Staphylococcus* infection, dermatophilosis), chorioptic mange, dermatophytosis, Malassezia infection, immune-mediated dermatitis (eg, pemphigus foliaceous) and neoplastic conditions (eg, sarcoids). Obtaining a complete history, thorough physical examination, skin scrapings, skin cytology, and biopsy of primary skin lesions early in the course of disease development may increase the likelihood of reaching a definitive diagnosis.

DIAGNOSIS

A detailed history is very important in the dermatologic work up of EPD.[5,8] Important pieces of information include age of onset, month of the year that problem was noted, and whether the EPD has been seasonal/nonseasonal or pruritic/nonpruritic. Additional questioning should include any overzealous use of topical medications or home remedies prior to the veterinarian's examination. Details should include what topical and systemic medications have been used and if lesions improved or worsened with each treatment. Environmental conditions can be a predisposing or primary factor in EPD, and when possible a detailed description or personal inspection of environment (bedding, pasture, sand, insect burden, moisture) should be done. Primary irritant and allergic contact dermatitis may involve the pastern region.[1,5,8,14] Chronic exposure to moisture such as wet bedding or muddy pastures appears to be the

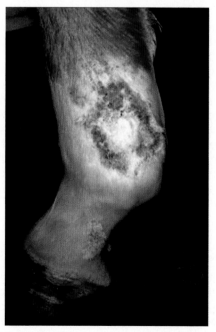

Fig. 6. PLV lesions consisting of well-demarcated circular painful, erythematous, exudative, tightly adherent crusts, typically involving nonpigmented areas of the legs and pasterns.

most common cause for irritant contact dermatitis. Draft horses have long hair in the fetlock and pastern region, which increases the retention of moisture and contributes to the maceration of the skin.[1,5,6,8]

Usually, in cases of contact irritant or allergic dermatitis, all 4 pasterns are affected. Be sure to ask whether other animals or people in contact with the affected horse are affected as well (infectious or zoonotic, ie, dermatophytes). Recurrences may also be related to the conformation of the food and pastern.[7]

Pastern folliculitis/pyoderma is caused by two main types of bacterial infections in the horse: *Staphylococcus aureus* and *Dermatophilus congolensis*.[1,6,8,14] Initially, papules and/or pustules (rare) will be noted with a *Staphylococcus* infection; however, with chronicity they may not be seen. A biopsy for culture would be needed for a definitive diagnosis. The area would need to be surgically scrubbed and biopsy taken with sterile precautions. Taking a swab of the area and culturing can be misleading because of surface contamination. *D congolensis* may also cause pastern dermatitis.[1,6,8,14,15] The lesions typically are crusting and exudative, and when crusts are removed, the skin is ulcerative.[16,17] Requirement for this organism to cause infection are chronic moisture and trauma.[15–17] A genetic susceptibility may exist. Immunocompromised and malnourished horses are far more susceptible, but serious infections can occur in almost any horse.[15] Immunity is short-lived, so recurrent infections may occur. Collection, staining, and microscopic examination for this organism will be described later in this article.

Dermatophytosis (*Trichophyton equinum*) rarely causes pastern folliculitis; however, it is important to rule out.[1,6,8,14] A definitive diagnosis requires a positive dermatophyte test media (DTM) culture in conjunction with positive microscopic identification of macrocondia.

Chorioptic mange may be the underlying cause of pastern dermatitis and must be excluded.[1,6,8,14,17,18] Draft horses are predisposed because of the long hairs over their pasterns.[5] This condition is intensely pruritic. Affected horses may constantly rub the area, and they often are observed stamping his feet.[5] This should be highly suspected if others in contact are affected and have clinical signs of pruritus. Mites are easily identified if infested.

Both systemic and contact forms of photosensitization may involve the pastern regions of the horse with white extremities.[19] When contact is involved, usually just the muzzle and extremities are involved. Primary photosensitization is due to a preformed or metabolically derived photosensitizing agent reaching the skin by ingestion, contact, or injection. Hepatogenous photosensitization is caused by blood phylloerythin levels that are elevated in association with liver abnormalities and a photodynamic agent.[5,19,20] Each type will cause dermatitis in the presence of UV light. The most common cause of equine contact photosensitization is exposure to clover pastures.[5] Other causes of primary photosensitization are Saint John's wort (*Hypericum perforatum*), buckwheat (*Polygonum fagopyrum*), and perennial rye grass (*Lolium perenne*).[19,20]

DIAGNOSTIC TESTS
Superficial Skin Scrape

Rule out superficial mites, especially *Chorioptes* subspecies. This can be done using a #10 blade (dull). Superficially scrape crusts and debris onto a slide. Others recommend using a stiff scrubbing brush or denture-type tooth brush to sweep the dander, crusts, and debris into a container.[4,18] Examine immediately under the microscope 10× objective, placing debris in mineral oil and using a cover slip. Some authors suggest applying a small amount of insecticide to the slide, because these mites are very fast.[21]

Adhesive Tape Impression + Diff Quik

Evaluate for secondary bacterial and Malassezia infections, which are often perpetuating factors. Observe under a microscope at 100× for cocci-shaped bacteria with or without degenerative neutrophils with intracellular and extracellular cocci and/or peanut-shaped purple yeast organisms.[6] The recommended tape is Scotch 3M Clear Packing Tape Pad (3M Center, St. Paul, MN), as its adhesive properties are stronger than the routine office tape, and it is more rigid, hence avoiding curling of the tape and making the dipping process more efficient. The sample should be collected and the tape stained with Diff Quik (Siemens Healthcare Diagnostics Inc., Deerfield, IL) (omitting the alcohol dip); one should then press it onto a glass slide and read it using a microscope. Acetate tape preps can also be used to identify *Chorioptes bovis*.[6,8,18]

Direct Examination of Hairs

Hair sampling to evaluate for dermatophytes is performed by plucking affected hairs with hemostat, placing them on a slide, and applying 1 to 2 drops of a clearing agent, 10% potassium hydroxide (KOH) solution, and applying a cover slip. Warm the slide for 15 to 20 minutes and evaluate hair shafts. First, under the 4× objective, search for infected hairs that appear pale and swollen. Second, re-examine under 40× for arthrospores within the hair shaft; these will appear as small clear bubbles in the hair shaft.[4,22] This is difficult as well as time-consuming and will take awhile to become experienced with this technique.

DTM Culture

When obtaining hair and crusts samples for a dermatophyte culture, one must add few drops of niacin (vitamin B complex) to all DTMs to satisfy the growth requirements of *Trichophyton equinum*, regardless of in-house culture or sending to laboratory. When preparing the site to take a culture, the use of isopropyl alcohol to cleanse the hairs of saprophytic (clinically irrelevant) fungi. It is important to allow the alcohol to dry prior to collection, or a false-negative result may be experienced. DTM will suppress growth of saprophytes and contaminant bacteria, because it contains chlorotetracycline, gentamycin, and cyclohexamide.[4,22,23] There is a phenol red pH indicator also included within the media. Dermatophytes use protein first, creating alkaline metabolites and red color change concurrently with colony growth. False-positive color changes occur; when saprophytes have exhausted the carbohydrate source on the plate, they will then utilize protein and cause a late red color change.[22] False-negatives occur (rarely). Once the red color change concurrent with colony growth is identified, microscopic examination is important to confirm the diagnosis. The procedure is as follows: typically 7 to 10 days of growth on the media are required before macroconidia are visualized. Use clear cellophane tape and press lightly onto the colony within the DTM. Then apply 1 to 2 drops of lactophenol cotton blue.[23] One may examine immediately under a microscope at 40×. If there are no macroconidia visible, wait a few days for the colony to mature and re-examine.

Dermatophilosis Congolensis Preparation

Place 1–2 drops of saline on a clean slide. Clip off excess hair from the crust sample and place crust into saline. Allow sample to macerate/soften for 15 minutes and then remove larger pieces. Crush out the remaining material on the slide and allow to air dry. Heat fix slide for a few seconds. Stain with Diff Quik or methylene blue. Allow to dry and examine under microscope 100X oil and with immersion you should visualize cocci shaped bacteria in a "railroad track" orientation.[4,23]

Biopsy for Histopathology

Biopsy should be considered if immune-mediated disorders or neoplastic conditions are suspected. Consideration of these differentials is also recommended when treatment has been pursued, and failures or relapses have occurred.[23] In most cases, especially a suspected, skin biopsies should be read out by a dermatohistopathologist with an interest in equine skin diseases.[6] Acute changes including leukocytoclastic vasculitis, thrombosis and vessel wall necrosis, are often scarce and can easily be overlooked; when present, they may provide a diagnosis.[5,6] Vessel wall thickening and hyalinization, along with epidermal hyperplasia or papillomatous, may be detected in chronic lesions. If secondary bacterial infection is severe, it is recommended to clear this before taking the biopsy.[23] For hyperplastic and nodular lesions, such as skin of severe CPL patients, a double punch biopsy is recommended, whereby a smaller 6 mm punch biopsy is introduced into the opening previously created by the skin sampled using an 8 mm biopsy. This technique will allow the practitioner to reach the deep dermis and subcutis for conditions such as CPL and panniculitis, respectively.

Biopsy for Culture

This may be necessary if bacterial or fungal infection is suspected or not responding to appropriate therapy.[18] When collecting a biopsy for culture, it is important to clip the hair and scrub the superficial area as if a surgical procedure were about to be performed. The biopsy is taken as sterile precautions are maintained and the sample placed in a sterile cup or sterile media. This should be sent to the laboratory as soon as possible. Otherwise, superficial contamination will compromise results.

Complete Blood Count and Chemistry Panel

These may useful in helping to rule out hepatogenous photosensitization disorders and other metabolic illnesses.[6]

Future Genetic Screening Tests

Mittman and colleagues[24] have identified quantitative trait loci (QTL) for CPL in 917 German draft horses. Thirty-one paternal half-sibling families comprising 378 horses from the breeds Rhenish German, Schleswig, Saxon-Thuringian (ECA9, 16, 17), and South German (ECA1,7) were recorded. This is an important step toward the generation of a screening test.

MEDICAL TREATMENTS

Choosing the appropriate therapy involves recognition and identification of predisposing, perpetuating, and primary factors.[6]

Environment

Recommendations include all of the following

1. Pastures and paddocks with mud, water or sand can predispose, and worsen the condition (ie, Arabian horses and sand).[1,6,8]
2. Keep horses in clean dry stalls during wet weather.
3. Do not release horses into pasture until the morning dew has dried.[6,8]
4. If contact allergy (affecting all pasterns) is suspected, suggest an alternate source of bedding (the treated or aromatic types of wood shavings contain chemicals that can cause contact hypersensitivity).[1,6,8,14]

5. If a horse has heavy hair feathers or has involvement around the ergot and at the back of the fetlock joint, clip feathers over the pasterns to decrease moisture retention.[1,6,8]
6. If PLV is suspected, avoid UV light exposure with stabling or wraps.[6,8,19,20]
7. The affected skin should be cleansed immediately after exercise while the sweat is still present using an antiseptic shampoo (eg, chlorhexidine).[25]
8. If lesions are located beneath the saddle, barrier creams prior to exercise, toweling or cotton sheet that is washed and changed daily may prevent further exacerbation of lesions.[25]
9. Lesions on the shoulders, blanket, and saddle pad contact zones should have a clean cotton or synthetic sheet as a barrier that can be washed on a regular basis.

Clinical Management—Topical Therapy Antibacterial

In EPD, secondary bacterial infections with *Staphylococcus* subspecies are a common problem that often complicates the diagnosis.[1,2,5,6] The antibacterial shampoos available are benzoyl peroxide 2%, ethyl lactate, or chlorhexidine 2%. Shampoo the area 1 to 2 times daily, lather, leave on 10 minutes, rinse, and dry well.[2,4–6] This should be done for 7 to 10 days, then to 2 to 3 times weekly. Another topical agent gaining increased use in both the human and veterinary fields is accelerated hydrogen peroxide (Pure Oxygen). This product can be applied to horses as a fungal wash/rinse or sprayed on and left to drip dry. It has an excellent spectrum of activity against various bacterial, fungal and viral pathogens (www.anivacfirst.com; www.virox.com) and is safe for use on all horses and surfaces.

Regardless of which topical agent is chosen, protection of the affected pastern(s) is imperative. Dry environment without bandaging is the most effective treatment. Some dermatologists recommend using a padded, water-repellent bandage (changed every 24–48 hours). Facilitator is a hydroxyethylated amylopectin liquid bandage that has been used successfully by some when applied every 1 to 3 days after cleansing.[2,6] If lesions are exudative, astringent solutions, such as lime sulfur or aluminum acetate solution, can be used. These agents will cause drying to the area and less exudation. Topical ointments are available for treating localized bacterial infections. Silver sulfadiazine and 2% mupirocin ointment both have excellent penetration into the epidermis and can be used for both dermatophilosis or staphylococcal infections.[2] Clipping and cleansing are paramount to success with any ointment.

Two recently studied additions to the topical armamentarium include Mudstop and kunzea ambigua oil (Greasy Heal KO). Ten of 11 cases treated with a Mud Stop (antibacterial agents and humectants, agents that lower water activity) revealed significant improvement.[26] In an Randomized Double Blinded Placebo Controlled (RDBPC) study, 7 days of kunzea oil topically resulted in complete resolution in 7 of 11 treated patients. Kunzea oil contains various active constituents such as pinene, 1–8-cineole (eucalyptol), and sesquiterpene alcohols. It is supplied as an ointment (20%) along with salicylic acid (50 g/kg) and reported to kill *S aureus* and various other gram-positive organisms, as well as yeasts and dermatophytes.[27]

Antifungal

Lime sulfur dips and spray can be used for localized treatment of the pastern for dermatophytes and mites. Enilconazole labeled for use in horses in many countries other than the United States and is used to treat fungal infections with good success.[2,6] Miconazole shampoo 1% or shampoo that contains miconazole 1% and chlorohexadine can be used.

Steroids

Topical steroids can be used for immune-mediated conditions such as PLV. Triamcinolone spray 0.015% and hydrocortisone 1% leave-on conditioner can be used in conjunction with systemic immunomodulators to treat this disease. In addition, good success has been noted with topical betamethasone 1% or aclometasone 0.05% applied to the lesion.[2] The author has recently had good success using mometasone (Mometamax) to treat PLV patients as part of a study protocol.

Systemic Therapy Antibiotic Medications

The most common antibiotic used in the horse is trimethoprim sulfamethoxazole (15–30 mg/kg every 12 hours). If the bacterial infection is severe, a 3-week course may be necessary, often in conjunction with topical antibacterial shampoos.[2,4,6,18] Monitor closely for signs of colitis/diarrhea and discontinue immediately if noted. Enrofloxacin 5 mg/kg of injectable orally every 24 hours has been used with success.[2,6] This drug should never be use in foals and growing horses. Procaine penicillin G -22,000 IU/kg intramuscularly twice daily for 7 to 10 days continues to be a reasonably priced injectable option for dermatophilosis.

Antifungal Medications

Systemic antifungal therapy is often unnecessary in the horse. Griseofulvin powder is available for the horse; however, there have been no pharmacokinetic data published, and the efficacy is questionable.[8,22] Ketoconazole, itraconazole, and fluconazole are effective for the systemic treatment of dermatophytosis in people, cats, and dogs. These agents are not currently approved for use in horses in the United States.[22] Ketoconazole (30 mg/kg) has very low absorption (23%) from the gastrointestinal tract in horses and can be expensive.[28] In addition, itraconazole and fluconazole can be used. The recommended dose for itraconazole is 5 to 10 mg/kg/d.[2,6,22,29] One published report using fluconazole in the horse recommends a loading dose of 14 mg/kg/d; then 5 mg/kg/d can be used safely.[30,31] The cost of these medications limits their use.

Immunosuppressive/Immunomodulary Therapy

Immune-mediated conditions such as PLV may need to be treated with immunosuppressive doses of steroids as well as decreasing the exposure to UV light.[2,5,6] Typically, dexamethasone, 0.1 to 0.2 mg/kg every 24 hours for 7 to 14 days, then tapered slowly over the next 4 to 6 weeks are recommended.[2,6] Prednisolone 2 mg/kg every 24 hours can be used also.[2,6] Pentoxifylline, 8–10 mg/kg every 12 hours by mouth, has immunomodulating properties such as inhibition of tumor necrosis factor (TNF)-α, interleukin (IL)-1, and IL-6. This drug has as been reported to be successful in a few cases. It is a phosphodiesterase inhibitor that increases red blood cell deformability and platelet aggregation, therefore inhibiting thrombosis. In addition, it influences leukocyte deformability and migration.[2,3] Long-term control can often be achieved using topical steroids and or pentoxifylline once the lesions are under control. An RDBPC study looking at the efficacy of pentoxifylline (Navicon) for treatment of PLV along with topical Mometamax is yielding promising results (Yu, personal communication, 2013).

Antiparasitic Therapy

Ivermectin (1% solution) should be given 300 μg/kg by mouth weekly for 4 doses.[2,4,6,21] To treat chorioptic mange, this may need to be repeated; treatment failures can occur, as these mites are surface feeders. A recent study in 19 horses looking at oral moxidectin (0.4 mg/kg body weight) given twice 3 weeks apart in combination with environmental treatment with 4-chloro-3-methylphenol and propoxur failed to yield positive results.[32] A prospective, double-blinded, placebo-controlled clinical trial found topical eprinomectin pour-on solution (at a dose of 500 μg/kg body weight weekly once for four applications) to be an effective and safe therapy against psoroptic mange infestation in hunter/jumper and dressage horses.[33] The author has used off-label eprinomectin with success to treat Chorioptes without any associated adverse events.

Although topical treatments are labor-intensive, they are currently the most effective. All contact animals and affected horses should be treated. Topical permethrin can be effective. Some authors suggest selenium sulfide shampoo followed by lime sulfur (6 oz/gallon), sponged on every 5 days for 1 month.[4,6,21] Fipronil spray 0.25% has been shown to be effective against Chorioptes bovis in 1 study.[18] These mites can live off the host up to 70 days, so environmental decontamination is important, including barn, stalls and bedding, tack, and grooming equipment.

SUMMARY

The prognosis of EPD depends on the underlying cause and the ability of veterinarians to identify it and the chronicity of the condition. Ensuring that predisposing, primary, and perpetuating factors are taken into consideration during the diagnostic work-up and treatment plan will optimize a positive outcome.

REFERENCES

1. Scott DW, Miller WH. Miscellaneous skin diseases. In: Scott DW, Miller WH, editors. Equine dermatology. London: Saunders; 2003. p. 687–90.
2. Yu AA. Pastern dermatitis. In: Robinson NE, editor. Current Therapy in Equine Medicine. 5th edition. Philadelphia, PA: WB Saunders; 2002. p. 201–3.
3. English M, Pollen S. Pastern dermatitis and unguilysis in 2 draft horses. Equine Pract 1995;17(8):25.
4. Logas DB, Barbet JL. Diseases of the skin. In: Colahan PT, Mayhew IG, Merritt AM, Moore JN, editors. Equine medicine and surgery. 5th edition. Goleta (CA): American Veterinary Publications; 1999. p. 1910–34.
5. Standard AA. Miscellaneous. Vet Dermatol 2000;11(3):217–23.
6. Akucewich L, Yu AA. Equine pastern dermatitis. In Compendium: Equine Edition 2007;2(4):214–28.
7. Pilsworth RC, Knottenbelt DC. Pastern and heel dermatitis. Equine Vet Educ 2006;18(2):93–5.
8. Ferraro GL. Pastern dermatitis in Shires and Clydesdales. J Equine Vet Sci 2001; 21:524–6.
9. de Cock HE, Affolter VK, Wisner ER, et al. Progressive swelling, hyperkeratosis, and fibrosis of distal limbs in Clydesdales, Shires, and Belgian draft horses, suggestive of primary lymphedema. Lymphat Res Biol 2003;1(3):191–9.
10. Available at: http://www.vetmed.ucdavis.edu/elephantitis/about.html. Accessed August 2013.
11. Powell H, Affolter VK. Combined decongestive therapy including equine manual lymph drainage to assist management of chronic progressive lymphoedema in draught horses. Equine Vet Educ 2012;24(2):81–9.
12. Pascoe RR, Knottenbelt DC. Pascoe. In: Manual of equine dermatology. London: WB Saunders; 1999. p. 165–6.

13. Risberg AI, Webb CB, Cooley AJ, et al. Leucocytoclastic vasculitis associated with Staphylococcus intermedius in the pastern of a horse. Vet Rec 2005; 156(23):740–3.
14. Pascoe RR, Knottenbelt DC. Iatrogenic or idiopathic disorders. Manual of equine dermatology. London: WB Saunders; 1999. p. 201–2.
15. Pilsworth RC, Knottenbelt D. Dermatophilosis (rain scald). Equine Vet Educ 2007; 19(4):212–4.
16. Scott DW, Miller WH. Bacterial skin diseases. In: Scott DW, Miller WH, editors. Equine dermatology. London: Saunders; 2003. p. 234–42, 13.
17. Pascoe RR, Knottenbelt DC. Manual of equine dermatology. London: WB Saunders; 1999.
18. Littlewood JD. Dermatosis of the equine distal limb. Proceedings of the 4th World Congress of Veterinary Dermatology. 2000. p. 129–33.
19. Rosenkrantz WS. Photo-induced dermatitis-vasculitis in the horse. 19th Proceedings of the AAVD & ACVD Annual Meeting. 2004. p. 123–7.
20. Boord M. Photosensitivity. In: Robinson NE, editor. Current Therapy in Equine Medicine. 5th edition. Philadelphia, PA: WB Saunders; 2002. p. 174–6.
21. Scott DW, Miller WH. Parasitic diseases. In: Scott DW, Miller WH, editors. Equine dermatology. London: Saunders; 2003. p. 331–3.
22. Scott DW, Miller WH. Fungal skin diseases. In: Scott DW, Miller WH, editors. Equine dermatology. London: Saunders; 2003. p. 261–76.
23. Scott DW, Miller WH. Diagnostic methods. In: Scott DW, Miller WH, editors. Equine dermatology. London: Saunders; 2003. p. 91–8.
24. Mittmann EH, Mömke S, Distl O, et al. Whole-genome scan identifies quantitative trait loci for chronic pastern dermatitis in German draft horses. Mamm Genome 2010;21(1–2):95–103.
25. Pilsworth RC, Knottenbelt D. Bacterial folliculitis. Equine Vet Educ 2007;19(6): 324–5.
26. Colles CM, Colles KM, Galpin JR. Equine pastern dermatitis. Equine Vet Educ 2010;22(11):566–70.
27. Thomas J, Narkowicz C, Peterson GM, et al. Randomised controlled trial of the treatment of pastern dermatitis with a formulation containing kunzea oil. Vet Rec 2009;164(20):619–23.
28. Prades M, Brown MP, Gronwall R, et al. Body fluid and endometrial concentrations of Ketoconazole in mares after intravenous injection or repeated lavage. Equine Vet J 1989;21(3):211–4.
29. Korenek NL, Legendre AM, Andrews FM, et al. Treatment of mycotic rhinitis with Itraconazole in 3 horses. J Vet Intern Med 1994;8(3):224–7.
30. Latimer FG, Colitz CM, Campbell NB, et al. Pharmacokinetics of Fluconazole following intravenous and oral administration and body fluid concentrations of Fluconazole following repeated oral doses in horses. Am J Vet Res 2001; 62(10):1606–11.
31. Scott DW, Miller WH. Dermatologic therapy. In: Scott DW, Miller WH, editors. Equine dermatology. London: Saunders; 2003. p. 189.
32. Rufenacht S, Roosje PJ, Sager H, et al. Combined moxidectin and environmental therapy do not eliminate Chorioptes bovis infestation in heavily feathered horses. Vet Dermatol 2010;22:17–23.
33. Ural K, Ulutas B, Kar S. Eprinomectin treatment of psoroptic mange in hunter/jumper and dressage horses: a prospective, randomized, double-blinded, placebo-controlled clinical trial. Vet Parasitol 2008;156(3-4):353–7.

Chronic Progressive Lymphedema in Draft Horses

Verena K. Affolter, Dr. med vet., Diplomate ECVP, PhD

KEYWORDS

- Lymphedema • Draft horses • Legs • Combined decongestive therapy
- Compression bandages • *Chorioptes bovis*

KEY POINTS

- Chronic progressive lymphedema (CPL) is an ultimately debilitating condition in draft horses.
- Although no permanent treatment is known, diligent management can improve the horses' conditions and prolong their use and life.
- Several factors contribute to this process.
- The high incidence within affected breeds highlights the importance of identifying underlying genetic factors in order to have a fair chance of winning the battle against CPL.

INTRODUCTION

Chronic progressive lymphedema (CPL) is a disabling disorder of many draft horse breeds, including Shires, Clydesdales, Belgian draft horses, Gypsy Vanners, English Cobs, several German draft horse breeds, and Friesians.[1–4] It also has been observed in Percherons in Europe. The clinical presentation resembles primary lymphedema in humans, also referred to as elephantiasis verrucosa nostra.[5–8] The clinical manifestations, etiopathogenesis, diagnostics, and therapies for primary lymphedema in humans have been addressed in several publications.

The horses present with progressive swelling of the distal portions of their legs, which is associated with scaling, marked dermal fibrosis, and the development of skin folds and nodules.[1] Typically, secondary recurrent bacterial and parasitic infections complicate these lesions and contribute to the aggravation of the lymphedema.[4] CPL is likely a multifactorial process with an underlying genetic component. It results in marked disfigurement of the distal extremities and, as such, often leads to lameness and premature euthanasia. Chronic progressive lymphedema has often erroneously been referred to as "chronic pastern dermatitis". The use of this term is discouraged,

The author has nothing to disclose.
Department of Pathology, Microbiology and Immunology, School of Veterinary Medicine, University of California, 3313 Vet Med 3A, Davis, CA 95616, USA
E-mail address: vkaffolter@ucdavis.edu

http://dx.doi.org/10.1016/j.cveq.2013.08.007
0749-0739/13/$ – see front matter
vetequine.theclinics.com

as it does not take into consideration that the inflammatory changes are secondary to the underlying disturbed lymph drainage. The clinical manifestations, etiopathogenesis, diagnostics, and therapies for CPL have also been addressed in several publications.

CAUSE AND PATHOGENESIS

The exact cause of equine CPL still needs to be elucidated.[6–11] Several studies indicate an altered elastin metabolism that results in an impaired function of the lymphatic system in the distal extremities. Given the high incidence of CPL in certain breeds, a genetic component likely contributes to the development of CPL. Several studies have elucidated that various additional factors contribute to the development of CPL. In summary:

1. Radiographs identify the soft tissue folds and nodules **(Fig. 1)**.
2. Lymphangiography illustrates the tortuous and dilated lymphatic vessels in legs of horses with CPL **(Fig. 2)**.[1]
3. Lymphoscintigraphy reveals significant accumulation of interstitial fluid and a slower clearance of a particular radiopharmaceutical in legs of horses with CPL, when compared with normal horses **(Fig. 3)**.[12]
4. The amino acid desmosine cross-links elastin fibers; its concentration in tissues reflects the amount of elastin. Desmosine within the skin of the neck and distal legs of clinically healthy horses of affected breeds are decreased when compared with other breeds.[13] Once the lesions develop the levels increase.[13]
5. Although elastin levels are generally low in the skin of healthy horses of affected breeds, the clinical lesions are mostly limited to the legs. Occasionally, there may be slight folding of the skin in the neck region. Hydrostatic pressure is considered an important contributing factor to the edema in the distal legs.[13] A higher risk for microtrauma and infections in this area enhances the lymphedema.

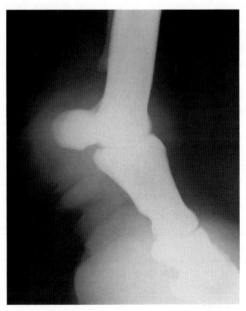

Fig. 1. Radiograph of the lower leg in a horse with CPL identifying the marked soft tissue swelling and formation of folds.

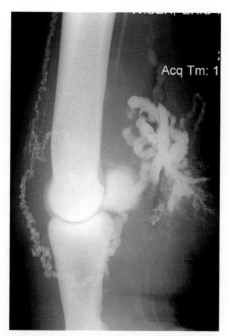

Fig. 2. Lymphangiography of a horse with severe CPL showing tortuous and dilated lymphatic vessels in the distal leg. (*From* De Cock HE, Affolter VK, Wisner ER, et al. Progressive swelling, hyperkeratosis, and fibrosis of distal limbs in Clydesdales, Shires, and Belgian draft horses, suggestive of primary lymphedema. Lymphat Res Biol 2003;3:193; with permission.)

6. Elastin repair and regeneration in adult tissues tends to result in a visually and functionally inappropriate fiber network.[10,14,15] The altered elastin network in affected horses can be visualized with special stains (acid-orcein Giemsa) or by immunohistochemistry using antielastin antibodies.[1,16] There is an increase of morphologically altered elastin fibers in a prominent disturbed arrangement within the superficial and middermis of affected horses when compared with clinically normal horses of affected breeds and horses of other breeds (**Fig. 4**). Dermal lymphatic vessels lack the normal concentric ring of elastin fibers observed in nonaffected breeds (**Fig. 5**).[1,16]

7. Horses with CPL have higher circulating antielastin antibody levels compared with clinically normal Belgian draft horses or healthy Warmblood horses.[17] This indicates tissue damage. Correlation of antibody levels with severity of disease is controversial.[17,18]

8. The high incidence of CPL and the challenge to find unaffected middle-aged or older horses within these breeds clearly indicates a genetic background to this disorder. In Belgian draft horses, CPL occurs after prolonged selected breeding with emphasis for dense feathering and heavier legs; this further suggests a genetic background for CPL. Moreover, certain familial lines of draft horses are more affected than other lines. The genetic predisposition of equine CPL, however, has not been characterized to date. None of the studies have identified a specific genetic marker and or mutation correlated with CPL. The studies performed to date include (1) forkhead transcription factor 2 gene (FOXC2)[19]

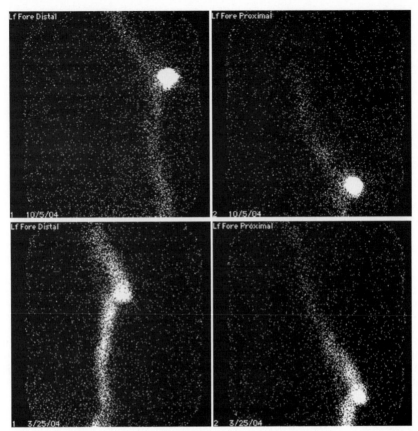

Fig. 3. Lymphoscintigraphy of the distal (*left*) and proximal (*right*) leg. Areas of external activity are added at the level of the accessory carpal bone as an anatomic reference point. In a normal horse there is weak to moderate staining of the contrast media left 30 minutes after injections (*top*) in comparison with a horse with mild CPL (*bottom*). (*From* De Cock HE, Affolter VK, Wisner ER, et al. Lymphoscintigraphy of draught horses with chronic progressive lymphoedema. Equine Vet J 2006;38:150; with permission.)

associated with primary lymphedema and distichiasis in humans, (2) ATP-ase Ca++316-transporting cardiac muscle slow twitch 2 isoform 2 gene (*ATP2A2*) associated with autosomal dominant inherited Darier-White disease, characterized by warty proliferations.[20,21] Four different quantitative trait loci were identified in the German draft horse. Some candidate genes were suggested within four different quantitative loci, but further studies are required.

9. Recurrent and persistent bacterial (*Staphylococcus* sp and *Dermatophilus congolensis*) and/or parasitic (*Chorioptes bovis*) infections are a typical event in horses with CPL.[1–4,22] Similar to primary lymphedema in humans, equine CPL is characterized by impaired circulation and lymph drainage.[7,8] This results in impaired skin barrier function and impaired function of the skin immune system. In addition, the heavy feathering leads to an occlusive environment supporting bacterial growth. With each bout of infection and inflammation, the lymph flow is increasingly impaired similar to the situation in humans with primary lymphedema.

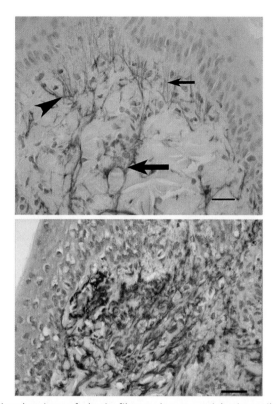

Fig. 4. Immunohistochemistry of elastin fibers using an antielastin antibody (NCL-Elastin, Novocastra, Illinois, USA) and diaminobenzidine as chromogen. Normal dermal elastin network (*top*) is characterized by oxytalan fibers (*small arrow*), the elaunin plexus (*arrowhead*) and the elastic fibers (*broad arrow*). The dermal elastin network of a horse with marked CPL (*bottom*) is disturbed; a dense band of clumped, distorted, and thickened elastin fibers is observed. (*From* De Cock HE, Van Brantegem L, Affolter VK, et al. Quantitative and qualitative evaluation of dermal elastin of draught horses with chronic progressive lymphoedema. J Comp Pathol 2009;140:136–7; with permission.)

10. The epidermal keratinocytes of lesional skin have altered expressions of cytokeratin 5, 6, 4, 10, and 14.[3] Increasingly evident in severe lesions, it is more consistent with a secondary phenomenon rather than the cause of the secondary infections.
11. Environmental factors influence the severity of CPL. With clean rubber flooring the lesions can be better controlled when compared with a sandy or muddy environment. Horses with regular exercise and turn out are less severely affected.

CLINICAL PRESENTATION

The lesions of CPL tend to be more pronounced in the hind legs, but both front and hind limbs can be affected.[1–4] Clinical signs become more evident as disease progresses. The presence of secondary infections markedly enhances the associated skin lesions. **Table 1** summarizes lesions observed and their correlation with severity of disease.

Mild and/or Early CPL

It is very difficult to palpate the early, mild thickening of the legs because heavy feathering obscures the early pitting edema. As a result, early signs of edema and mild

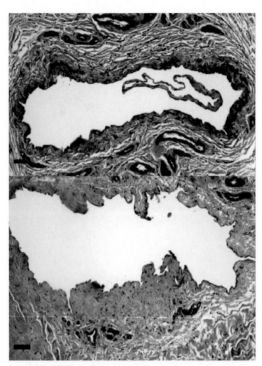

Fig. 5. Elastin network around lymphatic vessels of the deep soft tissues in a normal horse (*top*) using acid-orcein Giemsa. The concentric elastin network is missing in this lymphatic vessel of a horse with CPL (*bottom*). (*From* De Cock HE, Affolter VK, Wisner ER, et al. Progressive swelling, hyperkeratosis, and fibrosis of distal limbs in Clydesdales, Shires, and Belgian draft horses, suggestive of primary lymphedema. Lymphat Res Biol 2003;3:197; with permission.)

hyperkeratosis remain unnoticed. However, careful palpation can identify the lack of clear definition of the cannon bone, flexor tendons, and fetlock. Small ripples, a preliminary sign of subsequent skin folds, can be detected in horses as young as 2 years of age. The skin surface is scaly and often slightly greasy. Clipping of the feathering allows for the detection of early pitting edema and mild skin rippling, in particular in the fetlock and pastern areas (**Fig. 6**). Typically, owners become aware of the lesions at times of secondary parasitic and/or bacterial infections. Leg stomping and scratching associated with chorioptic mange, as well as oozing and crusting due to bacterial infections, initiate the more careful evaluations of the skin hidden below the dense feathering. Each bout of infection and inflammation will further disrupt lymph flow and increase the lymphedema.[1–4]

Moderate to Severe Chronic CPL

Typically, the lower extremities become more cone-shaped as clear definition of the cannon bone, flexor tendons, and the fetlock joint contours are lost. Prolonged pitting edema results in fibrosis of the skin and subcutis. As a result, the swollen, enlarged legs palpate as being very firm. The progressing fibrosis further impairs lymph flow. In addition to the increased circumference, the number, size, and depth of folds and nodules increases and may measure up to several centimeters (**Fig. 7**). This is

Table 1
Guidelines to categorize clinical evaluation of CPL using palpation and visual evaluation of skin surface; contour of lower legs; and presence of folds, nodules, and signs of secondary infection

Mild CPL	Moderate	Severe	Extreme
Slight skin thickening	Moderate skin thickening	Severe skin thickening	Severe skin thickening
Scaling	Prominent scaling	Severe scaling	Severe scaling
Pitting edema	Exudate, possible erosions, ulcers	Marked exudation, erosions, ulcers	Marked exudation, erosions, ulcers
Normal limb diameter	Increased leg diameter	Increased limb diameter	Feathering broken
Leg definition slightly blurred	Cone shape of lower leg	Firm swelling (brawny edema)	Large limb diameter
1–2 small folds of the pastern (P and PL)	Firm swelling (brawny edema)	Complete lack of leg definition	Firm swelling (brawny edema)
	Multiple folds, nodules in pastern and fetlock (D, P, PL)	Multiple skin folds, nodules ascending toward carpus or tarsus (D, P, PL)	Complete lack of leg definition extending above carpus, tarsus
		Possible mechanical disturbances	Numerous skin folds, nodules ascending to and above carpus or tarsus; circumferential
			Folds and nodules alopecic and ulcerated
			Severe mechanical impairment
			Possible secondary lymphangitis
Slight skin thickening			
Scaling			
Pitting edema			
Normal limb diameter			
Leg definition slightly blurred			
1–2 small folds of the pastern (P and PL)			

Abbreviations: D, dorsal; P, palmar; PL, plantar.

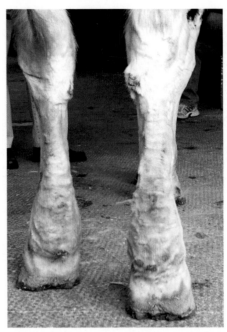

Fig. 6. Gypsy Vanner mare, 6 years old, with mild CPL. After clipping the feathering, it is evident that there is swelling of the pasterns, fetlocks, and lower areas of the cannon bones resulting in a slight cone shape of the lower extremity. The skin is slightly rippled and there are small folds in the pastern.

most evident in the palmar and plantar area of the pastern region, but extends proximally to the fetlock and, eventually, up to carpus and tarsus (**Fig. 8**).[1–4]

The skin surface is extremely scaly, often moist, and occasionally greasy. Unattended legs routinely have evidence of secondary infections: staphylococcal species

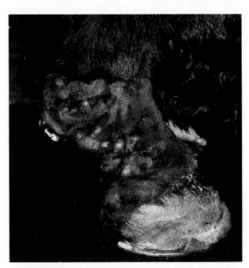

Fig. 7. Friesian mare, 8 years old, with moderate CPL. In addition to the swelling of the lower extremity, there are numerous firm skin nodules and folds, some of them eroded and ulcerated.

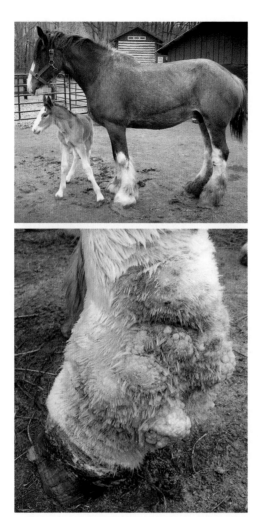

Fig. 8. Clydesdale mare, 13 years old, with severe CPL (*top*). The feathers are clumped and partially blood stained from the oozing skin lesions and both hind legs are swollen to the hock joints. Milder discoloration of the feathers is seen on the palmar region of both front legs and the swelling of the pastern area is still hidden by the feathering. After clipping of the feathers, the hind legs (*bottom*) reveal severe swelling, thick folds, and nodules with markedly irritated, erythematous skin surfaces. The coronary band is irregular and bulging.

and/or *C bovis* mites are the most common pathogens observed. Occasionally, *D congolensis* or other bacteria are isolated from the lesions. *C bovis* infections elicit marked pruritus, clinically evidenced by stomping the feet or rubbing the legs.

Many nodules, folds, and (occasionally) the skin in between become eroded and ulcerated (**Fig. 9**), either due to the trauma induced by constant scratching, interference with the gait, and/or impaired tissue perfusion.

By the time owners become overly concerned about the changes, the lesions have significantly progressed. The lesions may not be only pruritic but also painful, and many horses become very reluctant to have their legs touched. The periods between recurrent infections become shorter due to severely impaired lymph drainage and

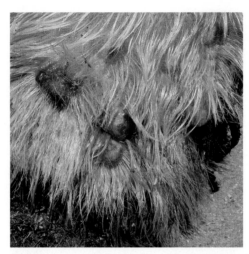

Fig. 9. Shire, 13 years old, with severe CPL. The fibrotic nodules are ulcerated.

tissue perfusion. Despite appropriate antibiotic and antiparasitic therapy, the erosions and the chronic dermatitis persist. The skin surface oozes, bleeds, and is covered with crusts. Persistent infections may affect deeper tissues and induce lymphangitis and swelling of the entire leg. The deep skin folds with the oozing surface are ideal niches for maggot infestation.

Associated Lesions of the Hooves

The coronary band is markedly hyperkeratotic and hyperplastic, which results in broad and deformed hooves of poor quality. The hoof walls are brittle and chipped with splits and cracks. Repeated bouts of thrush and deep hoof abscesses are commonly seen, and some horses develop laminitis.

Ergots and Chestnuts

Usually, CPL-affected horses have irregular, misshapen chestnuts and ergots.

HISTOPATHOLOGY

Diagnostic morphologic lesions are typically seen in hematyoxylin-eosin stained tissue sections of the deep dermis and subcutis.[1] The markedly dilated lymphatics are surrounded by edematous connective tissue that, eventually, transition to severe fibrosis (**Fig. 10**). There are increased numbers of vascular structures. For instance, many arteries have increased numbers of vasa vasorum (see **Fig. 10**). Mild inflammation may surround the lymphatics and vessels. Within the dense fibrosis, there may be encapsulated small abscesses. The inflammation may progress in to the deeper tissues and be associated with lymphangitis. The morphologic changes of superficial biopsy specimens tend to have lesser diagnostic value. There is marked acanthosis and hyperkeratosis. Intraepidermal pustules, erosions, ulcerations, crusts, and luminal folliculitis are observed with secondary infections (see **Fig. 10**). There may be micro-hemorrhage due to compromised vascular walls.

Acid-orcein Giemsa stains highlight the disturbed elastin network within the superficial dermis. The large, dilated lymphatics in the deeper tissues lack the supportive circular elastin network (see **Fig. 5**).[1,4]

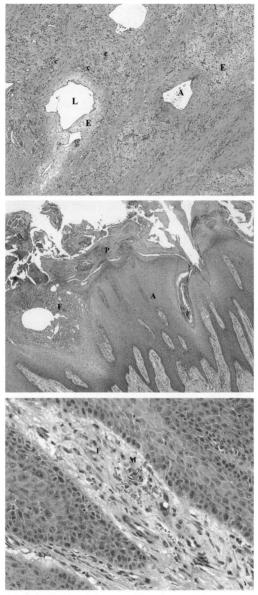

Fig. 10. Histology of skin with CPL. H&E staining. Deep dermis (*top*) of affected horse is characterized by dilated lymphatic vessels (L) with marked subacute edema with early fibrosis (E), increased numbers of small capillaries (C) and occasional arterial wall hyperplasia (A). Secondary infections (*middle*) is associated with a marked acanthosis (A), a thick layer of parakeratosis (P) and a pustule in the infundibular area of the follicle, indicating superficial folliculitis (F). The superficial dermis (*bottom*) may have variable degrees of fibrosis (F) and microhemorrhage (M) indicating vascular wall compromise.

Immunohistochemistry with antielastin antibodies illustrates the disarray of the elastin network (see **Fig. 4**) and the lack of perilymphatic elastin.[4,16]

DIAGNOSIS

The clinical presentation is very diagnostic, particularly in advanced stages. Thorough palpation of the lower extremity is necessary to recognize the early stages of the disease. Often, clipping of the feathers is mandatory to identify the extent of the lesions. If the owner is reluctant to clip the feathers, radiographs can be used to outline clearly the marked soft tissue swelling and folds along with identifying underlying bone and joint lesions. Lymphangiograms illustrate the markedly dilated, tortuous lymphatics in the distal legs. Lymphoscintigraphy ultimately confirms the diagnosis of impaired lymph drainage.[1,12] Although these are effective diagnostic methods to identify even the early stages of the disease, both are not readily available and are very expensive.

Thorough and repetitive skin scraping and tape tests may be necessary to identify *C. bovis* mites. With persistent infections, culture and sensitivity testing is recommended. Regular skin punch biopsies may not always be helpful because diagnostic changes from the deep dermis and subcutis may not be represented. A double-punch biopsy technique is often more rewarding and illustrates the changes of lymphatic vessels and vasculature. The first step in this biopsy technique uses an 8 mm punch through superficial and middermal epidermis. The second step involves driving a 6 mm punch through the previous 8 mm biopsy site to harvest the deep dermis and subcutis.

Diagnostic threshold values of circulating antielastin antibodies have not been broadly established. In the initial study, a correlation between levels of circulating antibodies and severity of lesions was observed.[17] This could not be validated in a subsequent study.[18] Hence, ELISA will likely not offer a reliable screening tool for presence and severity of CPL.

Genetic studies to develop reliable diagnostic screening tests have been unrewarding to date.[19–21]

MANAGEMENT

It is important that owners understand that they are dealing with labor-intesive symptomatic management of a life-long disease and that there is no successful permanent treatment.[23–25] Lesions progress, even if secondary bacterial infections and mite infestations are treated appropriately. Diligent daily care, however, can drastically improve the condition, slow down progression, and help avoid recurrent infections.

The most crucial first step to successful management is clipping the feathers and keeping hairs short. Initially, owners tend to oppose this suggestion vigorously. Therefore, it is important to explain that the extent of the lesions hidden below the feathers can only be assessed accurately after removal of the feathering. Moreover, this will allow access to the skin surface for appropriate topical treatment. Owners can be reassured that feathering can grow back to original lengths in 10 to 12 months.

Treatment of Bacterial Infections

Topical treatment starts with careful, gentle washing (without scrubbing) and drying of the legs. Nonirritating sulfur-based shampoos are recommended. Blow-drying may be required to dry the skin surface completely. Bacterial infections of deep skin folds can be managed with topical antimicrobials. The periodic changing of antimicrobials and correct treatment is important to avoid the development of microbial resistance. With severe bacterial skin infections and evidence of possible lymphangitis systemic antibiotic therapy is indicated.[2]

Treatment of Chorioptic Mange

Topical application of fipronil spray (Frontline, Merial Limited, Duluth, GA, USA) has been used successfully to treat *C bovis* mite infestations. Its use in horses has not been approved by the Food and Drug Administration. It should also be avoided in pregnant and lactating mares. Lime sulfur has also been routinely used for treatment of *C bovis* mites. It is an economical and effective topical treatment and is safe to use in pregnant mares. Wettable sulfur powder ("flowers of sulfur") can be mixed with mineral oil to form a creamy paste and applied to the affected areas. Frequent topical or systemic macrocyclic lactone treatment (eg, eprinomectin, ivermectin) helps prevent reinfestation with mites.[2,26–28]

Environment

To help prevent constant reinfestation with mites, pesticide applications in barns may be necessary. Affected horses need to be kept in a dry environment to avoid prolonged wet and muddy skin.

Daily Exercise and Skin Care

The importance of exercise must be emphasized because it increases circulation as well as lymph flow. Light exercise can be performed with compression bandages. See later discussion on combined decongestive therapy (CDT).

Daily Skin Care

Any irritation to the skin surface must be avoided because it enhances the lymphedema. The use of drying soaps, alcohol, and vigorous scrubbing are contraindicated. Nonirritating sulfur-based shampoos can be used on a regular basis. Keeping the feathers short assists in maintaining cleanliness of the skin surface. Moreover, it is easier to identify new secondary infections earlier. Cold-water rinses are recommended on legs with clipped feathers, in particular after exercise. However, it is important to dry the legs carefully after each rinse. A blow dryer can be used, especially if the feathering is growing back.

Hydrotherapy

A special whirlpool has been designed to treat horses in Belgium (www. paardenjacuzzi.com). In addition to having a cleaning effect, the hydrotherapy will further enhance blood circulation. After treatment, the legs need to be dried very carefully and the horses should be kept on dry clean surfaces for a few hours to ensure complete drying of hair coat and skin surface. It has to be emphasized that the Jacuzzi could potentially harbor bacteria if not meticulously cleaned after each treatment, which, together with the whirling effect, could result in skin infections.

Hoof Care

Routine foot trimming is essential because the hoof quality of horses with CPL is often impaired. Simultaneously, the ergots and chestnuts should be trimmed regularly, if necessary. Any inflammatory state enhances the progression of lymphedema. Daily careful hoof cleaning is important to address any flares of thrush immediately.

CDT

Combined decongestive therapy (CDT) is the most successful treatment of lymphedema in humans. In horses, this is achieved with a two-phase treatment plan that should be performed and overseen by an appropriately trained person. The treatment includes manual lymph drainage (MLD) and compression bandaging. MLD supports and stimulates the lymphatic system to move accumulated proteins and water from the interstitium back to the circulation. The goal is to move lymph in a "transterritorial" fashion from affected areas to areas where the lymphatic system is functioning adequately. In addition, MLD induces breakdown of indurated fibrotic tissue, which is most prominent within the nodules and folds. Clipping the feathers will make the treatment considerably more effective. For subsequent compression, specialized multilayer short-stretch bandages (eg, Rosidal, Lohmann & Rauscher International GmbH & Co KG, Topeka, KS, USA and Wien, Austria) are applied over carefully padded limbs. The short-stretch bandages create a pressure gradient up the leg.[28–30]

Phase I of CDT

In phase I, daily MLD is followed by immediate specialized multilayer compression bandaging. Keeping bandages applied 24 hours per day and for at least 7 days of the week coincides with the best results. Light exercise such as walking is highly recommended while bandages are left on (**Fig. 11**). The massaging effect of the short stretch bandages during light exercise reduces the edema and swelling. During the early phases of this therapy, the lymphedema will ooze through the skin. This necessitates daily bandage changes. The skin needs to be dried, MLD repeated, and the compression bandage reapplied. This daily routine is repeated until no further reduction of the leg circumference, nodules, and folds is observed and the skin surface has improved.

Phase II of CDT

Phase II is the long-term management of the disease. Skin care is continued. Horses can go back to their regular exercise program. It is important to maintain an appropriate exercise program to support good circulation and lymph drainage. Specialized knitted cotton compression garments (Kerstin Gutberlet Strumpfproduktion u. Handel, Burghbaun, Germany) for horses are available to avoid prompt recurrence of the lymphedema (**Fig. 12**). Occasional, lymph drainage treatments can be applied as needed.

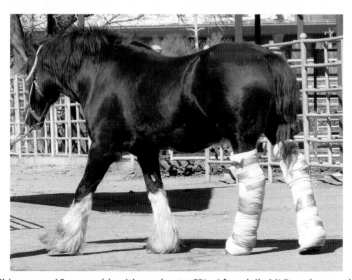

Fig. 11. Shire mare, 16 years old, with moderate CPL. After daily MLD and correctly applied compression bandaging, the mare is hand-walked (light exercise). During movement, the compression bandage has a massaging effect and assists in the movement of lymph from the lower legs back into the circulation.

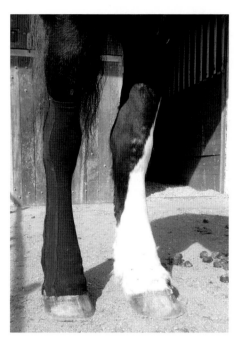

Fig. 12. Shire mare, 16 years old, with moderate CPL. After completing the phase 1 of the CDT, which includes MLD and subsequent compression bandaging, compression garments (Kerstin Gutberlet Strumpfproduktion u. Handel, Burghbaun, Germany) is used to keep the recurrence of the edema under control.

Surgical Approach with Postsurgical Pressure Bandaging

Similar to techniques used in humans with lymphedema, surgical debulking of nodules or epidermal shaving with subsequent compression bandaging have been described as possible interventions for horses with CPL. However, each surgical intervention will disrupt the lymphatic vascular bed that is already challenged. Moreover, development of exuberant granulation tissue secondary to large wounds in lower extremities is a well-recognized sequela and therapeutic challenge in horses. Therefore, surgical intervention is not highly recommended.[31,32]

SUMMARY

CPL is an ultimately debilitating condition in draft horses. Although no permanent treatment is known, diligent management can certainly improve a horse's condition and prolong its use and life. The high incidence within affected breeds highlights the importance of identifying underlying genetic factors in order to have a fair chance of winning the battle against CPL.

REFERENCES

LYMPHEDEMA IN HUMANS

1. Cheville AL, McGarvey CL, Petrek JA, et al. Lymphedema management. Semin Radiat Oncol 2003;13:290–301.
2. Daroczy J. Pathology of lymphedema. Clin Dermatol 1995;13:433–44.

3. Földi E, Földi M, Weissleder H. Conservative treatment of lymphoedema of 523 the limbs. Angiology 1985;36:171–80.
4. Frances C, Robert L. Elastin and elastic fibers in normal and pathological skin. Int J Dermatol 1984;3:166–79.
5. Gerli R, Ibba L, Fruschelli C. A fibrillar elastic apparatus around human lymph capillaries. Anat Embryol 1990;181:281–6.
6. Harwood CA, Mortimer PS. Causes and clinical manifestations of lymphatic failure. Clin Dermatol 1995;13:459–72.
7. Koul R, Dufan T, Russell C, et al. Efficacy of complete decongestive therapy and manual lymphatic drainage on treatment-related lymphedema in breast cancer. Int J Radiat Oncol Biol Phys 2007;67:841–6.
8. MacLaren JA. Skin changes in lymphoedema: pathophysiology and management options. Int J Palliat Nurs 2001;7:381–8.
9. Richards RN. Verrucous and elephantoid lymphedema: morphologic spectrum and terminology. Int J Dermatol 1981;20:177–87.
10. Skobe M, Detmar M. Structure, function, and molecular control of the skin lymphatic system. J Investig Dermatol Symp Proc 2000;5:14–9.
11. Vaccaro M, Borgia F, Guarneri F, et al. Elephantiasis nostras verrucosa. Int J Dermatol 2000;39:760–73.

LYMPHEDEMA IN DRAFT HORSES

12. De Cock HE, Affolter VK, Wisner ER, et al. Progressive swelling, hyperkeratosis, and fibrosis of distal limbs in Clydesdales, Shires, and Belgian draft horses, suggestive of primary lymphedema. Lymphat Res Biol 2003;3:191–9.
13. De Cock HE, Affolter VK, Wisner ER, et al. Lymphoscintigraphy of draught horses with chronic progressive lymphoedema. Equine Vet J 2006;38:148–51.
14. De Cock HE, Affolter VK, Farver TB, et al. Measurements of skin desmosine as an indicator of altered cutaneous elastin in draft horses with chronic progressive lymphedema. Lymphat Res Biol 2006;4:67–72.
15. De Cock HE, Van Brantegem L, Affolter VK, et al. Quantitative and qualitative evaluation of dermal elastin of draught horses with chronic progressive lymphoedema. J Comp Pathol 2009;140:132–9.
16. De Keyser K, Oosterlinck M, Raes E, et al. Early detection of chronic progressive lymphedema susceptibility in Belgian draught horse stallions by means of ELISA. Commun Agric Appl Biol Sci 2012;77:183–7.
17. Fedele C, von Rautenfeld DB. Manual lymph drainage for equine lymphoedema-treatment and therapist training. Equine Vet Educ 2007;19:26–31.
18. Ferraro G. Chronic progressive lymphedema in draft horses. J Equine Vet Sci 2003;23:189–90.
19. Geburek F, Ohnesorge B, Deegen E, et al. Alterations of epidermal proliferation and cytokeratin expression in skin biopsies from heavy draught horses with chronic pastern dermatitis. Vet Dermatol 2005;16:373–84.
20. Harland MM, Fedele C, Berens v Rautenfeld D. The presence of myofibroblasts, smooth muscle cells and elastic fibers in the lymphatic collectors of horses. Lymphology 2004;37:190–8.
21. Littlewood JD, Rose JF, Paterson S. Oral ivermectin paste for the treatment of chorioptic mange in horses. Vet Rec 1995;137:661–3.
22. Mittmann EH, Momke S, Distl O. Whole-genome scan identifies quantitative trait loci for chronic pastern dermatitis in German draft horses. Mamm Genome 2010;21:95–103.

23. Momke S, Distl O. Molecular genetic analysis of the ATP2A2 gene as candidate for chronic pastern dermatitis in German draft horses. J Hered 2007;98:267–71.
24. Poore LA, Else RW, Licka TL. The clinical presentation and surgical treatment of verrucous dermatitis lesions in a draught horse. Vet Dermatol 2012;23:71–5.
25. Powell H, Affolter VK. Combined decongestive therapy including equine manual lymph drainage to assist management of chronic progressive lymphoedema in draught horses. Equine Vet Educ 2012;24:81–9.
26. Rötting AK. Manuelle Lymphdrainage - Erprobung an den Extremitäten des Pferdes. Thesis Anatomie der Medizinischen Hochschule Hannover and Klinik fur Pferde Chirurgie Freie Iniversität. Berlin, Germany, 1999. p. 135.
27. Rüfenacht S, Roosje PJ, Sager H, et al. Combined moxidectin and environmental therapy do not eliminate *Chorioptes bovis* infestation in heavily feathered horses. Vet Dermatol 2011;22:17–23.
28. Wallraf A. Populationsgenetische Untersuchung zum Aftreten 412 von Mauke bei den deutschen Kaltblutpferderassen [Inaugural Dissertation]. Hannover, Germany: Tierärztliche Hochschule Hannover; 2003. p. 144.
29. Van Brantegem L. Chronic progressive lymphedema in draught horses [Doctoral Thesis]. Gent, Belgium: University Antwerp and Gent; 2007. p. 133.
30. Van Brantegem L, DeCock HE, Affolter VK, et al. Antibodies to elastin peptides in sera of Belgian Draft horses with chronic progressive lymphedema. Equine Vet J 2007;39:418–21.
31. Vlamink L, De Cock HE, Hoesten H, et al. Epidermal shaving for hyperpapillomatosis secondary to chronic progressive lymphoedema in Belgian drafthorses. Vet Dermatol 2008;19S:76.
32. Young AE, Bower L, Affolter VK, et al. Evaluation of FOXC2 as a candidate gene for chronic progressive lymphedema in draft horses. Vet J 2007;174:397–9.

Immune-Mediated Dermatoses

Wayne Rosenkrantz, DVM

KEYWORDS

- Immune mediated • Autoimmune • Pemphigus • Lupus erythematosus
- Bullous pemphigoid • Erythema multiforme • Purpura hemorrhagica

KEY POINTS

- Pemphigus foliaceus is the most common autoimmune skin disease in the horse and is associated with the production of autoantibodies directed against surface proteins of the keratinocyte, which mediate intercellular adherence.
- Pemphigus vulgaris is a rare autoimmune skin disease in horses.
- Both systemic lupus erythematosus (SLE) and cutaneous lupus erythematosus (CLE) have been recognized in the horse and both conditions are extremely rare.
- Bullous pemphigoid is a rare autoimmune disease in horses, caused by immunologic attack of the basement membrane zone by autoantibodies.
- Erythema muliforme is an immunologic reaction in the skin in which keratinocyte cell death (apoptosis) is the prominent change seen on biopsy.
- Purpura hemorrhagica (PH) is thought to be analogous to nonthrombocytopenic purpura or Henoch-Schönlein purpura in humans.

INTRODUCTION

Immune-mediated dermatoses are commonly divided into primary (or autoimmune) and secondary (or immune-mediated diseases). In autoimmune diseases, antibodies or activated lymphocytes develop against normal body constituents. In immune-mediated diseases, the antigen is foreign to the body and may include drugs, bacteria, and viruses, which stimulate an immunologic reaction that results in host tissue damage. The problem with subdividing immune-mediated diseases into primary and secondary causes is that it is not always known if the antigen is foreign or not and what initially stimulates the self-destructive process. In some situations, "epitope spreading" occurs, wherein antibodies are formed against a foreign infectious protein initially but, as the disease evolves, additional antibodies are made against molecules that are similar in structure and can resemble or mimic a normal body or cellular antigen (mimicry). This article discusses pemphigus foliaceus and pemphigus vulgaris,

The author has nothing to disclose.
Animal Dermatology Clinic, 2965 Edinger Avenue, Tustin, CA 92780, USA
E-mail address: infotustin@adcmg.com

Vet Clin Equine 29 (2013) 607–613
http://dx.doi.org/10.1016/j.cveq.2013.08.001   vetequine.theclinics.com

bullous pemphigoid, lupus erythematosus, erythema multiforme (EM), and purpura hemorrhagica.

PEMPHIGUS FOLIACEUS

Pemphigus foliaceus is the most common autoimmune skin disease in the horse and is associated with the production of autoantibodies directed against surface proteins of the keratinocyte, which mediate intercellular adherence. These autoantibodies bind to the surface of the keratinocyte stimulating acantholysis. This disorder can wax and wane and is characterized clinically by the presence of vesicles and pustules. In the horse, finding primary pustules is rare because lesions rapidly progress to crusted erosions, which result in alopecia, scaling, and crusting. Alopecia, scaling, and crusting are the most common presenting findings. Pruritus, pain, edema, and fever are variable. Lesions may begin on the face or limbs and spread to the rest of the body. A localized form restricted to the coronary bands is also seen. Pemphigus is identified in both adults and young horses less than 1 year of age.[1,2] Younger horses often have a better prognosis for response and potential remission without further relapses. Although Appaloosas seemed at risk in initial case reviews,[2] more recent reviews do not support this finding.[1,3] Quarter horses and Thoroughbreds may be more predisposed.[1,3] In these more recent reviews, no gender predilections were found and 80% of the cases had the first onset of lesions between September and February.[1,3] This may reflect insect exposure or other preventative medicine practices (worming, vaccines, and so forth) used during specific times of the year. These recent reviews also support that the most common presenting signs are edema and crusting followed by pain, pruritus, and fever. In addition to the cutaneous clinical lesions, systemic signs may include depression, poor appetite, weight loss, and fever.[1,3]

Pemphigus foliaceus should be considered in all skin diseases that have scaling and crusting. Differential diagnoses should include dermatophytosis, dermatophilosis, systemic granulomatous disease, and primary keratinization disorders.

The presence of compatible clinical lesions, cytology, and skin biopsies is an important consideration when making the diagnosis of pemphigus foliaceus. Cytology can be taken from intact pustules or erosive-crusted lesions. Often, single or rafts of acantholytic cells are found on Wright or Diff-Quik staining. Generally few or no bacteria are found from intact pustules and only extracellular bacteria may be found from erosive, crusted samples. Optimally, biopsies should be taken from primary vesicles or pustules and should identify acantholytic cells. Intact pustules are rarely encountered. For this reason, taking biopsies from crusted sites is the next best choice. Such areas should not be surgically prepared because this can remove the crusts containing acantholytic cells, which deleteriously affects the diagnostic value of the biopsy. Direct immunofluorescence and immunohistochemistry testing should reveal a diffuse intercellular deposition of immunoglobulins IgG and IgM and occasionally complement within the epidermis. In one report, skin-fixed intercellular epidermal IgGs were found in most horses.[2] In the same report, indirect immunofluorescence testing revealed circulating antikeratinocyte autoantibodies in 5/9 (56%) horses with pemphigus foliaceus.[2] These additional tests are performed rarely in equine cases. Diagnostic emphasis is placed on routine histopathology. Other potential abnormal laboratory findings include mild normocytic normochromic anemia, neutrophilia, mild hypoalbuminemia, and hypergammaglobulinemia.

Treatment is usually accomplished by using high dosages of glucocorticoids. Prednisolone is preferred to prednisone in the horse due to the limited efficacy of prednisone in horses. This is related to its poor absorption and/or biotransformation into prednisolone.[4] Prednisolone is generally effective at high induction dosages for a 7- to 10-day period. Dosages range from 1.5 mg/kg to 2.5 mg/kg every 24 hours with tapering over several weeks. This is followed by a maintenance dosage of 0.5 mg/kg to 1 mg/kg every 48 hours. Occasionally, other forms of glucocorticoids may be needed. Dexamethasone is used, starting at dosages of 0.02 mg/kg to 0.1 mg/kg every 24 hours for 7 to 10 days, which is then tapered to 0.01 mg/kg to 0.02 mg/kg every 48 to 72 hours. Injectable gold salts have also been used successfully in horses with pemphigus foliaceus, specifically aurothioglucose (Solganal). Unfortunately this form of injectable gold salts is no longer available. An alternative injectable gold salt is auro-thiomalate (Myochrysine). In a protocol extrapolated from human literature, test doses of 20 mg and 50 mg are given at weekly intervals to evaluate for potential deleterious side effects, which include eosinophilia and cutaneous reactions. If no abnormal reactions are seen, then an induction maintenance dose is given. This is administered intramuscularly at 1 mg/kg weekly with a long lag phase of 6 to 12 weeks before response is seen. Monitoring for bone marrow suppression (in particular, thrombocytopenia), drug reactions, and proteinuria is recommended. There are reports in the literature using azathioprine at 1 mg/kg to 3 mg/kg every 24 to 48 hours for various autoimmune skin diseases in horses.[5,6] The potential side effects of using azathioprine are thrombocytopenia, leukopenia, and anemia, because horses have low levels of the enzyme, thiopurine methyltransferase,[7] which is responsible for the metabolization of azathioprine. The author has used azathioprine at 1 mg/kg to 3 mg/kg for 1 month, then every 48 hours in 2 horses with no deleterious effects. It is also used as a steroid-sparing drug, in an attempt to eventually decrease the steroid needed for long-term management. The use of azathioprine in horses may be cost prohibitive, however, for most clients. Other adjunctive agents that the author has tried with variable success include pentoxifylline (Trental) at 10-15 mg/kg every 12 hours and omega-3 and omega-6 fatty acids.

The management of pemphigus foliaceus requires patience and support on an owner's part. This disease can wax and wane and may take weeks to months to control. In younger horses, the response and prognosis is generally good, with some cases of complete remission without ongoing therapy. In adult horses, there is a small percentage of cases when control does not occur. In 1 retrospective study, 5 of 13 horses (38%) were euthanized for either lack of response to treatment or development of steroid-induced acute laminitis[1]; 4 of 11 horses (36%) remained in remission for more than 1 year after immunosuppression.[1] In another study, follow-up information was reported for 7 of 15 horses.[3] Only 1 horse was euthanized due to financial constraints, whereas the other horses achieved remission with prednisone, prednisolone, or aurothioglucose.[3] In 1 horse, long-term remission was maintained in the absence of treatment.[3]

PEMPHIGUS VULGARIS

Pemphigus vulgaris is a rare autoimmune skin disease in horses. Clinical signs include mucosal and periorificial ulceration, which may extend into the esophagus. Recently, a case report was confirmed of a 9-year-old Welsh pony stallion with both direct and indirect immunofluorescence and immunoprecipitation studies, the latter identifying circulating anti–desmoglein 3 IgG. Treatment with immunosuppressive medications was initiated. Lesions were seen in the perineal area, sheath, mane, tail, eyelids, coronary bands, and mucosa of the mouth and esophagus. Initial glucocorticoid treatment improved the clinical signs, but the onset of laminitis necessitated a reduction in dosage, which was associated with a recurrence of lesions and development of oral ulcers. A corneal ulcer developed after 60 days of treatment. Other drugs were added, including azathioprine, gold salts, and dapsone, but the disease progressed and the pony was euthanized. Post-mortem examination showed additional lesions at the cardia of the stomach.[8] Other reports also note that glucocorticoid therapy has not proved helpful in cases of pemphigus vulgaris.[9]

LUPUS ERYTHEMATOSUS

Both SLE and CLE have been recognized in the horse. Both conditions are extremely rare. CLE typically presents primarily as a facial pattern with erythema, alopecia, and depigmentation. Antinuclear antibody (ANA) testing is negative. Biopsy should show basal cell degeneration, pigmentary incontinence, apoptotic keratinocytes in the basal cell layer, and a lichenoid infiltrate; however, on occasion, healthy horses may normally have some basal cell degeneration and thickening of the basement membrane zone. One study showed that the prevalence of apoptotic keratinocytes was significantly greater (52%) in cases of discoid lupus erythematosus, EM, photodermatitis, and systemic lupus erythematosus than in other dermatoses (8%).[10]

SLE can present with generalized scaling, alopecia, and internal organ dysfunction. Diagnosis can be difficult but is usually made by biopsy (similar findings to CLE) and optimally meeting certain criteria as set forth by the revised 1982 American College of Rheumatology classifications, which includes a positive ANA test. Such criteria are often not met, however, even in human medicine. Making a diagnosis of SLE can be difficult and challenging.[11] Ultimately, the diagnosis of SLE is based on clinical findings and the evaluation of all organ systems with a complete blood cell count, serum diagnostic panel, and urinalysis. Glucocorticoids at immunosuppressive dosages are indicated (see previous discussion of pemphigus foliaceus). Topical glucocorticoids and topical 0.1% tacrolimus are also tried in more localized cases. SLE cases can be more difficult to treat and many horses are euthanized due to lack of response.[12]

BULLOUS PEMPHIGOID

Bullous pemphigoid is a rare autoimmune disease in horses, caused by immunologic attack of the basement membrane zone by autoantibodies. Clinical lesions include crusts and especially ulcers. Bullae are rare. Ulceration may involve the gastrointestinal tract. Although other species frequently have many eosinophils histologically, the horse does not. Bullous pemphigoid is characterized histologically by subepidermal cleft and vesicle formation. Acantholysis does not occur. Inflammatory infiltrates vary from mild to severe, with both perivascular and lichenoid patterns seen. Treatment is the same as that of pemphigus foliaceus, although the few cases seen or reported have not had favorable outcomes.[13] A paraneoplastic bullous stomatitis that resembled bullous pemphigoid has been reported but may have been a case of paraneoplastic pemphigus.[14]

ERYTHEMA MULTIFORME

EM is an immunologic reaction in the skin in which keratinocyte cell death (apoptosis) is the prominent change seen on biopsy. There are many possible etiologic factors, including infectious diseases, drugs, systemic disease, and neoplasia.[15] In horses, drugs are considered a potential cause. More recently, newer emphasis has been placed on possible viral causes. In humans, herpes simplex virus is responsible for precipitating most of the EM episodes in adults and children.[16] Recently a report of a facial pustular dermatitis in a horse was found associated with equine herpesvirus 5 (EHV-5), indicating that EHV-5 should be strongly considered as a cause of lympho-histiocytic interface dermatitis with intranuclear inclusion bodies in horses and has similarities to herpes-associated EM in humans.[17]

Unfortunately, the underlying causes of many cases of EM are not defined and the EM is termed idiopathic. EM is believed to be an immunologically mediated disorder in which keratinocytes may be targeted specifically by killer lymphocytes.

Clinical lesions are characterized by macules, papules, urticaria or vesicles, and bullae. Individual lesions may expand peripherally leading to the formation of target-like lesions. True target lesions as described in human EM have not been documented in horses. Scaling and crusting is usually not a feature of equine EM, unless the disease is initially characterized by erosions or ulcers. Individual lesions can persist for several days. Pruritus and pain are variable but usually are not seen. Lesions may occur in association with or after an infection, such as EHV-5 or drug administration. One notable researcher theorized that reticulated and hyperesthetic leukotrichia may also represent a form of EM in the horse.[9]

The diagnosis is based on history, physical examination, and optimally skin biopsies. The histologic changes are distinctive and often include an interface or a cytotoxic inflammatory pattern with keratinocyte apoptosis with lymphocyte satellitosis. Vesicular lesions may be present and can include more confluent areas of keratinocyte destruction with massive spongiosis and subepidermal or intraepidermal edema.

Differential diagnoses should include urticaria, amyloidosis, and other nodular or papular diseases. Treatment should be directed toward the underlying cause, if one can be found. Recent or past history of herpes virus should be checked. Drug history is also important. Although some cases of EM are self-limiting and may resolve within a 1- to 3-month period, trial courses of glucocorticoids at immunosuppressive dosages with or without pentoxifylline might be tried (see previous discussion of pemphigus foliaceus).

PURPURA HEMORRHAGICA

PH is thought analogous to nonthrombocytopenic purpura or Henoch-Schönlein purpura in humans.[18] It is considered a form of anaphylactoid purpura, which characteristically occurs in children in the spring of the year after an upper respiratory tract infection. The disease is essentially a severe necrotizing vasculitis with resulting purpuric lesions in the skin and mucous membranes, with larger hemorrhagic and edematous lesions in the muscle and subcutaneous tissues. When the latter occurs in affected horses, it can cause marked edema and stocking up of the limbs with lameness and stiffness. Thrombosis of intestinal vessels can lead to gastrointestinal bleeding, colic, and death. Icterus, fever, and severe depression can accompany the disease.

The usual cause of the disease in most horses is a *Streptococcus equi* infection involving the respiratory tract, often with abscessation at some internal site.[18] Alternatively, PH has also been associated with other causes, such as vaccines prepared from *S equi*. It is postulated that the streptococcal antigens precipitate an immunologic response by IgA antibodies.[19]

A large study of 53 cases of PH in horses attempted to characterize etiology, signalment, clinical lesions, clinopathology, and treatment outcome. Seventeen horses were exposed to or infected with *S equi* and 9 with *Corynebacterium pseudotuberculosis*, 5 had been vaccinated with *S equi* M protein, 5 had had a respiratory infection of unknown etiology, and 2 had open wounds. The other 15 cases had no history of recent viral or bacterial infection. Age of onset ranged from 0.6 to 19 years (mean 8.4 years). The predominant clinical signs were well-demarcated subcutaneous edema of all 4 limbs and hemorrhages on the visible mucous membranes; other signs included depression, anorexia, fever, tachycardia, tachypnea, reluctance to move, drainage from lymph nodes, exudation of serum from the skin, colic, epistaxis, and weight loss. Hematological and biochemical abnormalities commonly detected were anemia, neutrophilia, hyperproteinemia, hyperfibrinogenemia, hyperglobulinemia, and elevated muscle enzymes. All reported horses were treated with glucocorticoids; 42 also received nonsteroidal anti-inflammatory drugs and 26 received antimicrobial drugs. Selected horses received special nursing care, including hydrotherapy and bandaging of the limbs. Most of the horses were treated for more than 7 days and none of them relapsed. Forty-nine of the 53 horses survived, 1 died, and 3 were euthanized, due to secondary complications. Two of the 4 nonsurvivors had been vaccinated against S equi with a product containing the M protein, 1 had a S equi infection, and the other had a respiratory infection of undetermined etiology.[20]

REFERENCES

1. Vandenabeele SI, White SD, Affolter VK, et al. Pemphigus foliaceus in the horse: a retrospective study of 20 cases. Vet Dermatol 2004;15(6):381–8.
2. Scott DW, Walton DK, Slater MR, et al. Immune-mediated dermatoses in domestic animals: ten years after. Part I. Compend Cont Ed Pract 1987;9:424–35.
3. Zabel S, Mueller RS, Fieseler KV, et al. Review of 15 cases of pemphigus foliaceus in horses and a survey of the literature. Vet Rec 2005;157(17): 505–9.
4. Peroni DL, Stanley S, Kollias-Baker C, et al. Prednisone per os is likely to have limited efficacy in horses. Equine Vet J 2002;34(3):283–7.
5. Humber KA, Beech J, Cudd TA, et al. Azathioprine for treatment of immune-mediated thrombocytopenia in two horses. J Am Vet Med Assoc 1991;199(5): 591–4.
6. McGurrin MK, Arroyo LG, Bienzle D. Flow cytometric detection of platelet-bound antibody in three horses with immune-mediated thrombocytopenia. J Am Vet Med Assoc 2004;224(1):83–7, 53.
7. White SD, Maxwell LK, Szabo NJ, et al. Pharmacokinetics of azathioprine following single-dose intravenous and oral administration and effects of azathioprine following chronic oral administration in horses. Am J Vet Res 2005;66(9): 1578–83.
8. Winfield LD, White SD, Affolter VK, et al. Pemphigus vulgaris in a Welsh pony stallion: case report and demonstration of antidesmoglein autoantibodies. Vet Dermatol 2013;24(2):269–74.
9. Stannard A. Immunologic diseases. Vet Dermatol 2000;11(3):163–78.
10. Macleod KD, Scott DW, Erb HN. The prevalence of apoptotic keratinocytes in equine epidermis: a retrospective light-microscopic study of skin-biopsy specimens from 253 horses with normal skin or inflammatory dermatoses. J Vet Med A Physiol Pathol Clin Med 2004;51(9–10):400–4.
11. Hay EM. Systemic lupus erythematosus. Baillieres Clin Rheumatol 1995;9(3): 437–70.
12. Geor RJ, Clark EG, Haines DM, et al. Systemic lupus erythematosus in a filly. J Am Vet Med Assoc 1990;197(11):1489–92.

13. Olivry T, Borrillo AK, Xu L, et al. Equine bullous pemphigoid IgG autoantibodies target linear epitopes in the NC16A ectodomain of collagen XVII (BP180, BPAG2). Vet Immunol Immunopathol 2000;73(1):45–52.
14. Williams MA, Dowling PM, Angarano DW, et al. Paraneoplastic bullous stomatitis in a horse. J Am Vet Med Assoc 1995;207(3):331–4.
15. Marshall C. Erythema multiforme in two horses. J S Afr Vet Assoc 1991;62(3): 133–6.
16. Weston WL. Herpes-associated erythema multiforme. J Invest Dermatol 2005; 124(6):xv–xvi.
17. Herder V, Barsnick R, Walliser U, et al. Equid herpesvirus 5-associated dermatitis in a horse-Resembling herpes-associated erythema multiforme. Vet Microbiol 2010;155:420–4.
18. Kaese HJ, Valberg SJ, Hayden DW, et al. Infarctive purpura hemorrhagica in five horses. J Am Vet Med Assoc 2005;226(11):1893–8, 45.
19. Boyle A. Streptococcus equi subspecies equi Infection (Strangles) in Horses. Compend Contin Educ Vet 2010;33(3):E1–8.
20. Pusterla N, Watson JL, Affolter VK, et al. Purpura haemorrhagica in 53 horses. Vet Rec 2003;153(4):118–21.

Equine Sarcoidosis

Marianne M. Sloet van Oldruitenborgh-Oosterbaan, DVM, PhD[a],*,
Guy C.M. Grinwis, DVM, PhD[b]

KEYWORDS

- Equine • Horse • Sarcoidosis • Granuloma

KEY POINTS

- The prognosis of generalized and partially generalized ES is poor.
- The prognosis of localized ES is good with respect to survival but guarded for the localized skin problem because only 26.7% recovered fully after treatment and 53% needed continuous low-maintenance dose prednisolone that is given between 7.00 AM and 9.00 AM (0.2–0.5 mg/kg/d).
- Recognition of the different forms of sarcoidosis based on history, clinical appearance, and histopathology assists owners in making an informed choice between treatment and euthanasia, and prevents unnecessary (local) treatment strategies.
- Localized ES should always be considered in the differential diagnosis of a localized exfoliative dermatitis of unknown origin.

INTRODUCTION

Equine sarcoidosis (ES) has several other names, such as equine idiopathic granulomatous disease, equine generalized granulomatous disease, equine systemic granulomatous disease, equine histiocytic disease, and equine histiocytic dermatitis.[1–4] ES is a rare disease complex that may present as either an exfoliative dermatitis or as a nodular skin condition, which is characterized by granulomatous inflammation of multiple organs.[3–6]

INCIDENCE

Nowadays, ES seems to be a more frequently encountered problem in equine dermatology. The reason for this may be either a better recognition of the different appearances of sarcoidosis and/or a real increase in prevalence. Before 2004, most published studies described only one or two cases. In 2004, Loewenstein and

---

The authors have nothing to disclose.
[a] Department of Equine Sciences, Faculty of Veterinary Medicine, Utrecht University, Yalelaan 112, 3584 CM Utrecht, The Netherlands; [b] Department of Pathobiology, Faculty of Veterinary Medicine, Utrecht University, Yalelaan 1, 3584 CL Utrecht, The Netherlands
* Corresponding author.
E-mail address: m.sloet@uu.nl

colleagues[7] reported six cases collected over four continents. The author more recently described 15 and 22 cases in two separate reports.[5,6] There seems to be no evidence of seasonality associated with this condition.[4,6,8]

FORMS OF SARCOIDOSIS

Sarcoidosis can be categorized as generalized, partly generalized, and localized. In the former two presentations, peripheral lymphadenopathy may be noted.[3–6,9] The localized form tends to remain focused within the skin without systemic signs.[10] Horses with the partly generalized form usually progress to the generalized form.[6] Horses with the generalized form of ES may start with an exfoliative dermatitis or with granulomatous inflammatory nodules in multiple organs. Both forms have similar prognoses: horses with the exfoliative form almost invariably develop nodules, and horses with the nodular form usually develop a scaling and crusting dermatitis.[4–6] In a study of 22 cases, 14% showed the generalized form, 18% the partially generalized form, and 68% the localized form.[6] The localized form most often occurs on the lower aspects of either pigmented and/or nonpigmented limbs.[5,6] The onset of sarcoidosis may be insidious or rapid.[2,4,6] The various forms of the clinical presentation of sarcoidosis are seen in **Figs. 1–9**.

CLINICAL SYMPTOMS

No age or gender predilections have been documented.[2–5] Sarcoidosis has been described as early as 3 months of age.[3,7] However, most horses are older than 3 years of age.[5,6,8,11–14] This observation is also consistent with the occurrence in humans, where the disease is also very rare in children.[15] The authors have found the disease

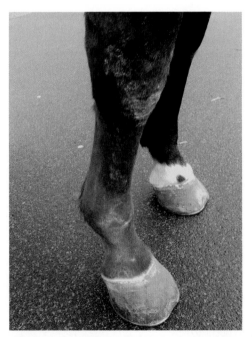

Fig. 1. Localized sarcoidosis on the right forelimb in an 8-year-old Dutch Warmblood mare with crusting, scaling, and hair loss of more than a year's duration.

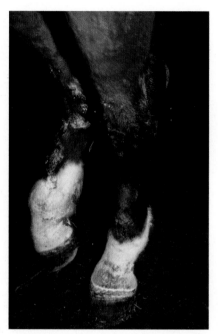

Fig. 2. Localized sarcoidosis of both hind limbs in a 16-year-old Dutch Warmblood gelding with crusting, scaling, and hair loss of more than a year's duration.

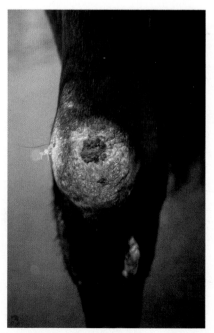

Fig. 3. Detail of the patient in **Fig. 2**. Both hocks were involved and also showed secondary lesions.

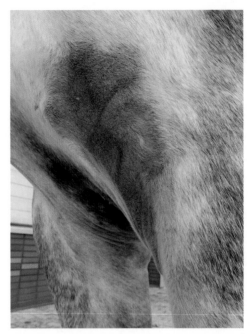

Fig. 4. Lateral view of partly generalized sarcoidosis in a 12-year-old Dutch Warmblood mare with exfoliative dermatitis on the chest and the left forelimb and some cutaneous nodules on the chest.

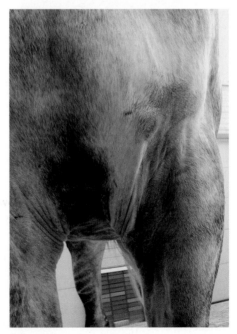

Fig. 5. Anterior view of the patient shown in **Fig. 4**.

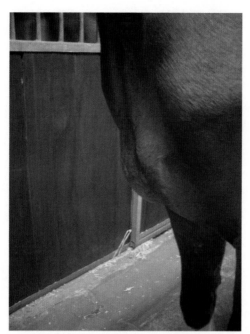

Fig. 6. The chest of a 7-year-old Dutch Warmblood gelding with generalized nodular sarcoidosis. The horse had several smaller and larger nodules all over the body. At first these were all covered with normal skin. Later some developed crusting of the overlying skin.

to be more prevalent in mares (63%) than in male horses (37%).[6] This is in accordance with the findings in humans, where women have a higher rate of sarcoidosis than men.[15]

ES has been reported to occur in many different breeds, including Warmbloods, Friesians, Arabians, standardbreds, thorougbreds, and ponies.[3,4,6,8] Two reports noted a predisposition for thoroughbreds and geldings.[7,8]

The skin lesions are characterized by focal, multifocal, or generalized extensive scaling and crusting with varying degrees of alopecia and increased local skin temperature. Lesions may occur all over the body, although most lesions are seen on the lower limbs.[2–6] Lesions are often discretely demarcated.[3]

In cases of the generalized nodular form, subcutaneous edema accompanies the nodule formation.[6] Internally, nodules may be found in order of decreasing frequency in the lungs, lymph nodes, liver, gastrointestinal tract, spleen, kidneys, bones, and central nervous system.[2–4,6,16] In some generalized cases of sarcoidosis, cutaneous involvement may not be present.[14,16] Most generalized sarcoidosis cases progress to a wasting syndrome characterized by one or more of the following signs: exercise intolerance, increased resting respiratory rate, mild dyspnea, poor appetite, weight loss, ventral edema, and persistent or fluctuating low-grade fever.[2,4,6,16] In contrast to human sarcoidosis, pruritus is rarely encountered in ES.[3,4,6,8,12,17]

ETIOLOGY

There is no proved etiology or causative agent, although many have been suggested.[2–4] In humans, it is believed that sarcoidosis may be an aberrant reaction to an infectious agent or antigen and this may also be true in the horse.[2,8,9,15] Spiegel and colleagues[8] could not identify any infectious causative agent and these authors

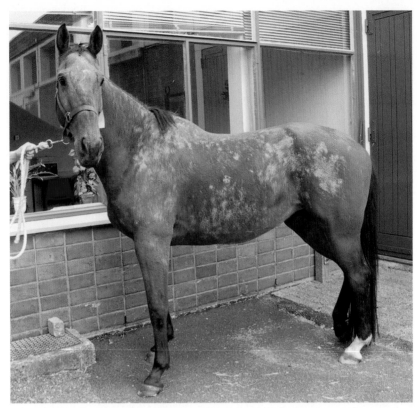

Fig. 7. Generalized cutaneous sarcoidosis with extensive skin lesions over the whole body in a 12-year-old Trakehner mare. There were no lesions at the mucocutaneous junctions.

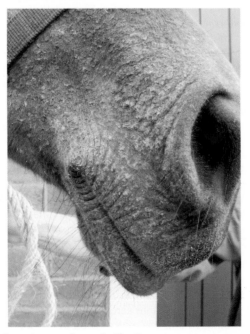

Fig. 8. Detail of the horse's nose shown in **Fig. 7**.

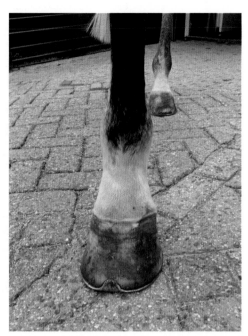

Fig. 9. A 6-year-old Dutch Warmblood mare with skin problems of the left forelimb of 6 months' duration. The skin is thickened and shows some crusts and some alopecia. The coronet and hoof wall are also abnormal. The limb is slightly painful and warm. This is an example of a mixed form of sarcoidosis and lower-limb vascultitis. (*Courtesy of* Jessica Bakker, DVM).

concluded that ES is unlikely to have a microbial etiology. Although White and colleagues[18] reported that they failed to detect DNA from equine herpesviruses 1 and 2 in paraffin-embedded skin of eight ES cases, they concluded that their findings did not discount equine herpesviruses 1 or 2 as a cause of some cases of ES. A putative causative role for *Mycobacterium* spp in the pathogenesis of ES, as has been proposed for human sarcoidosis, was suggested in a single equine case.[13] The absence of any identifiable causative mechanism means that the disease continues to be a diagnosis by exclusion.[8]

HISTOPATHOLOGY

The diagnosis of cutaneous ES is confirmed by skin biopsy. Histologic evaluation of cutaneous ES is characterized by multifocal nodular to diffuse, lymphogranulomatous dermatitis with multinucleated giant cells. A vasculitis may also be present.[6] The histologic appearance of ES is depicted in **Figs. 10–17**.

THERAPY

Most authors suggest that corticosteroids are the therapy of choice[2,4,6,19] and include the following:

- An initial high dose of systemic corticosteroid (prednisolone at 1–2 mg/kg orally once daily followed by a lower dose of prednisolone [0.20–1 mg/kg orally once daily]) for several weeks or longer.

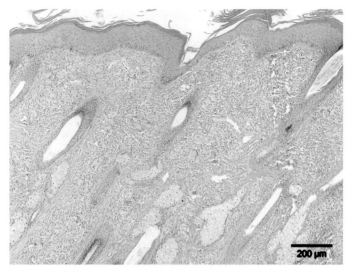

Fig. 10. Skin biopsy of the mare in **Fig. 1** revealed a marked lymphohistiocytic dermatitis with multinucleated Langhans-type giant cells (hematoxylin and eosin).

- Dexamethasone at 0.04–0.08 mg/kg intramuscularly once daily for 7 to 14 days and followed by prednisolone.
- All glucocorticosteroid treatments are given between 7:00 AM and 9:00 AM to support the endogenous day-night rhythm of cortisone.
- No local treatment is advised because the skin of affected areas is, in most cases, already fragile and sensitive.

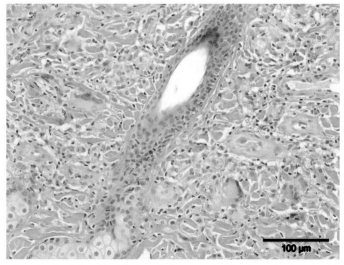

Fig. 11. Further detail of the skin biopsy of the mare in **Fig. 1**, again showing the multinucleated giant cells (hematoxylin and eosin).

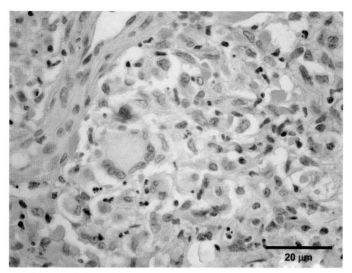

Fig. 12. A skin biopsy of the gelding in **Fig. 2** showed lymphohistiocytic infiltrates and a multinucleated Langhans-type giant cell (hematoxylin and eosin).

In addition to corticosteroids, dietary omega 6/omega 3 fatty acids may also be used for at least 3 to 12 weeks (dosage depending on manufacturer). Tumor necrosis factor-α inhibitors, such as pentoxifylline, have been shown to be beneficial in refractory human sarcoidosis cases.[15] Pentoxifylline given at 10 mg/kg twice daily orally may be used as an adjunct to steroids but the benefits of these are not established in ES.[4] Dietary changes may be helpful because diseases similar or identical to ES have been caused in field cases by hairy vetch (*Vincia velosa*).[3,20]

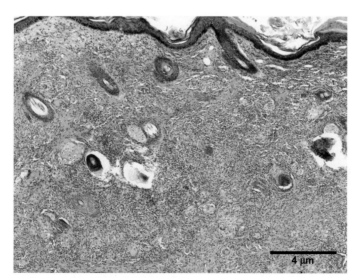

Fig. 13. Skin biopsy of the patient shown in **Figs. 4** and **5** revealed marked lymphohistiocytic infiltrates in the dermis and scattered Langhans-type multinucleated giant cells (hematoxylin and eosin).

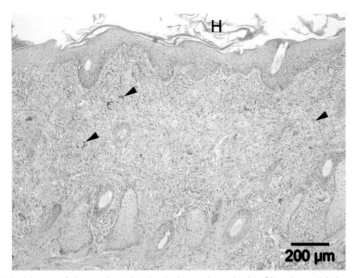

Fig. 14. Skin biopsy of the patient in **Fig. 6** showed marked infiltration with lymphocytes, histiocytes, and Langhans-type multinucleated giant cells (*arrowheads*) (hematoxylin and eosin).

PROGNOSIS

The prognosis of generalized sarcoidosis is poor.[1,5,6,12] However, some authors describe that weight gain may occur during corticosteroid therapy and that euthanasia may not be required.[21] The prognosis for the partially generalized form is also poor, although this may be related to the type of owner.[6] Spontaneous resolution has also been reported in the generalized form and in the localized form.[2,4–6] The prognosis

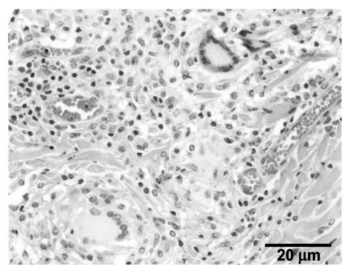

Fig. 15. Skin biopsy of the patient shown in **Figs. 7** and **8** revealed several Langhans-type giant cells with abundant pale eosinophilic cytoplasm and a rim of peripheral nuclei (hematoxylin and eosin).

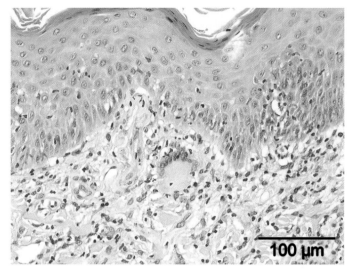

Fig. 16. A skin biopsy of the patient shown in **Fig. 9** shows features of sarcoidosis (lymphohistiocytic infiltrates and Langhans-type multinucleated giant cells) and of vasculitis (thickened blood vessel walls) (hematoxylin and eosin).

for the localized form seems to be good for survival but guarded with respect to the localized skin problem. These observations are highlighted in a previous report of nine patients diagnosed with localized sarcoidosis (four geldings and five mares, 5–20 years of age) wherein two of nine horses with localized sarcoidosis fully recovered, whereas seven of nine showed some improvement, but significant disease persisted.[10] These results are also compatible with the prognosis for 22 cases of localized sarcoidosis more recently compiled by the author.[6] However, in that study several

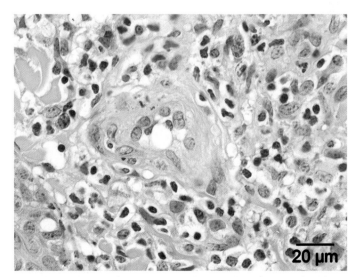

Fig. 17. A more detailed view of **Fig. 16** showed marked thickening of a blood vessel wall with presence of nuclear debris within the wall (hematoxylin and eosin).

horses were euthanized or slaughtered because the skin problem did not resolve and the owner did not want a horse that required continuous medication. These cases were therefore not able to contribute to knowledge of the natural course of the disease.

In some of the equine patients with localized sarcoidosis, concurrent vasculitis has been seen. There is no explanation for this phenomenon. This association might be an expression of a common underlying immune-mediated mechanism.

SUMMARY

ES seems to be an emerging problem. As more horses are referred for dermatologic disease, ES should be considered in any case of exfoliative and/or a nodular skin disease with or without systemic involvement. With the present knowledge of equine sarcoidosis, it can be stated that

- The prognosis of generalized and partially generalized ES is poor.
- The prognosis of localized ES is good with respect to survival but guarded for the localized skin problem because only 26.7% recovered fully after treatment and 53% needed continuous low-maintenance doses of prednisolone that is given between 7.00 AM and 9.00 AM (0.2–0.5 mg/kg/d).
- Recognition of the different forms of sarcoidosis based on history, clinical appearance, and histopathology assists owners in making an informed choice between treatment and euthanasia and prevents unnecessary (local) treatment strategies.
- Localized ES should always be considered in the differential diagnosis of a localized exfoliative dermatitis of unknown origin.

REFERENCES

1. Heath SE, Bell RJ, Clark EG, et al. Idiopathic granulomatous disease involving the skin in a horse. J Am Vet Med Assoc 1990;197:1033–6.
2. Stannard AA. Systemic granulomatous disease. Vet Dermatol 2000;11:170–2.
3. Knottenbelt DC. Sarcoidosis (generalized granulomatous disease). In: Knottenbelt DC, editor. Pascoe's principles and practice of equine dermatology. 2nd edition. Edinburgh: Saunders Elsevier; 2009. p. 280–1.
4. Scott DW, Miller WH. Sarcoidosis. In: Scott DW, Miller WH, editors. Equine dermatology. 2nd edition. Missouri: Elsevier Saunders; 2011. p. 453–5.
5. Sloet van Oldruitenborgh-Oosterbaan MM, Koeman JP. Recognition and therapy of sarcoidosis. In: Proceedings of the 45th Annual Congress of the British Equine Vet Association. 2006. 184–5.
6. Sloet van Oldruitenborgh-Oosterbaan MM, Grinwis GC. Equine sarcoidosis: clinical signs, diagnosis, treatment and outcome of 22 cases. Vet Dermatol 2013;24: 218–24.e48.
7. Loewenstein C, Bettenay SV, Mueller RS. A retrospective study of equine sarcoidosis. Vet Dermatol 2004;15:67.
8. Spiegel IB, White SD, Foley JE, et al. A retrospective study of cutaneous equine sarcoidosis and its potential infectious aetiological agents. Vet Dermatol 2006;17: 51–62.
9. Fadok VA. An overview of equine dermatoses characterized by scaling and crusting. Vet Clin North Am Equine Pract 1995;11:43–51.
10. Sloet van Oldruitenborgh-Oosterbaan MM, Koeman JP. Equine sarcoidosis: a systemic disease or a localised dermatosis? In: Proceedings of the 41st Annual Congress of the British Equine Vet Association. 2002. 210–11.

11. Axon JE, Robinson P, Lucas J. Generalised granulomatous disease in a horse. Aust Vet J 2004;82:48–51.
12. Hansmann F, Venner M, Hewicker-Trautwein M, et al. Sarkoidose bei einer Warmblutstute. Tierärztliche Praxis Grosstiere 2007;5:363–8.
13. Oliveira-Filho JP, Monteiro LN, Delfiol DJ, et al. *Mycobacterium* DNA detection in liver and skin of a horse with generalized sarcoidosis. J Vet Diagn Invest 2012;24: 596–600.
14. Peters M, Graf G, Pohlenz J. Idiopathic systemic granulomatous disease with encephalitis in a horse. J Vet Med A Physiol Pathol Clin Med 2003;50:108–12.
15. Haimovic A, Sanchez M, Judson MA, et al. Sarcoidosis: a comprehensive review and update for the dermatologist. J Am Acad Dermatol 2012;66:699.e1–18.
16. Reijerkerk EP, Veldhuis Kroeze EJ, Sloet van Oldruitenborgh-Oosterbaan MM. Generalized sarcoidosis in two horses. Tijdschr Diergeneeskd 2008;133:654–61.
17. Goldberg A, Lang A, Mekori YA. Prolonged generalized pruritus associated with selective elevation of IgA as the presenting symptoms of sarcoidosis. Ann Allergy Asthma Immunol 1995;74:387–9.
18. White SD, Foley JE, Spiegel IB, et al. Lack of detectable equine Herpesviruses 1 and 2 in paraffin-embedded specimens of equine sarcoidosis. J Vet Intern Med 2009;23:623–5.
19. Schlipf JW Jr. Dermatological conditions associated with crusts and scales: sarcoidosis. In: Robinson NE, editor. Current therapy in equine medicine. 4th edition. Philadelphia: WB Saunders; 1997. p. 384.
20. Woods LW, Johnson B, Hietala SK, et al. Systemic granulomatous disease in a horse grazing pasture containing vetch (*Vicia* sp.). J Vet Diagn Invest 1992;4: 356–60.
21. Rose JF, Littlewood JD, Smith K, et al. A series of four cases of generalized granulomatous disease in the horse. In: Kwochka KK, Willemse T, von Tscharner C, editors. Advances in Veterinary Dermatology: Proceedings of the 3rd World Congress Veterinary Dermatology, Edinburgh, Scotland, September 11–14, 1996.

Noninflammatory, Nonpruritic Alopecia of Horses

Rod A.W. Rosychuk, DVM

KEYWORDS

- Equine • Alopecia • Alopecia areata • Telogen effluvium • Follicular dysplasia
- Trichorrhexis

KEY POINTS

- Non inflammatory, non pruritic alopecias are uncommon in the horse.
- Telogen effluvium and alopecia areata are the most commonly seen.
- The performance of a thorough history and dermatologic examination alone often leads to a presumptive diagnosis for several of these problems.
- When the diagnosis is not clear, trichograms and skin biopsies can provide valuable insight. Maximal value from skin biopsies is associated with taking multiple samples.

NONINFLAMMATORY, NONPRURITIC ALOPECIA

The list of differential diagnoses for alopecia in the horse is long (**Box 1**). Most are related to inflammatory or pruritic diseases. Noninflammatory, nonpruritic dermatoses are relatively uncommon. Most are only anecdotally reported and lack substantial study data. Although these problems are clinically noninflammatory, their pathogenesis may involve follicular inflammation (eg, alopecia areata, linear alopecia). Within this group, alopecia areata is the entity that is encountered most frequently and has been most thoroughly evaluated. It is discussed in greatest detail.

The diagnosis of most of these alopecias is based on history, physical examination, trichography, and skin biopsies. Skin biopsies should ideally be taken from areas that are most significantly alopecic, the margins of alopecic areas, more recently developing lesions, and adjacent more normally haired areas. Emphasis is placed on taking larger samples (eg, 8-mm punch biopsies) and multiple biopsies (at least 3 or 4 or more). This allows for histologic evaluation of larger numbers of hair follicle units. Biopsies should be accompanied by a thorough history, a description of lesions and ideally submitted.

The author has nothing to disclose.
Department of Clinical Sciences, Colorado State University, 300 West Drake, Fort Collins, CO 80523, USA
E-mail address: rrosychu@colostate.edu

Vet Clin Equine 29 (2013) 629–641
http://dx.doi.org/10.1016/j.cveq.2013.09.005

Box 1
Equine alopecia

A. Congenital alopecia

    1. Congenital hypotrichosis[a]

B. Acquired alopecia

Noncicatrichial alopecia: hair regrowth occurs if causative factors are eliminated or corrected

1. Trauma (pruritus/self-trauma)

2. Altered hair follicle function

    a. Telogen effluvium[a]

    b. Anagen effluvium[a]

    c. Seasonal alopecia[a]

    d. Hypothyroidism[a]

    e. Color dilution alopecia[a]

    f. Follicular dysplasia[a]

    g. Protein, copper, or iodine deficiency[a]

    h. Chemical toxicosis: selenosis, arsenic, mercury, mimosine[a]

3. Defects in hair shafts

    a. Trichorrhexis nodosa[a]

    b. Piedra[a]

4. Inflammation of the hair follicle (folliculitis/furunculosis)

    a. Bacterial pyoderma

    b. Dermatophytosis

    c. Alopecia areata[a]

    d. Linear alopecia[a]

Cicatrichial alopecia: permanent destruction of hair follicles; regrowth does not occur

1. Physical, chemical or thermal injury

2. Severe furunculosis

3. Neoplasia

4. Cutaneous onchocerciasis

  [a] Clinically noninflammatory, nonpruritic alopecias.
Modified from Stannard AA. Alopecia in the horse – an overview. Vet Dermatol 2000;11:191; with permission.

Alopecia Areata

Alopecia areata is an uncommonly encountered disease in the horse and is also seen in humans, primates, dogs, cats, cattle, poultry, mice, and rats.[1,2] Its pathogenesis has been more thoroughly studied in only 1 horse.[3] As in other species, it seems to be an autoimmune disease in which IgG autoantibodies are directed at specific antigens of anagen (growing) hair follicles. These antigens are within the inner and outer root sheath and precortex of the lower aspects of the follicle and include trichohyalin and other keratins.[3] Antibodies targeting these regions of the hair follicle associated with growth and differentiation are suspected to disrupt follicle function. IgG from an affected horse that had high circulating IgG antibodies to hair follicle antigens induced follicle telogenization and prevented hair regrowth when injected into normal black mice.[3] Lymphocytes accumulate around the follicle and within the follicular root sheaths of the deeper portions of the hair follicle (up to the isthmus of the follicle) and within the hair bulb of anagen hairs (bulbitis). Intrabulbar lymphocytes are more frequently CD8+ (cytotoxic).[4] Follicles subsequently go into the catagen and telogen (resting) phases of the hair cycle. They may atrophy and become dysplastic (abnormal shapes/contours) and may contain dysplastic hair shafts. Follicles may become miniaturized, although this finding is more controversial.[5] With chronicity, the inflammatory component of the process wanes and may essentially disappear, leaving only dysplastic follicles. Although the earlier phases of this disease are histologically inflammatory, on a clinical basis only hair loss is noted; inflammatory changes are not seen.

There is a genetic predisposition to this disease in both mice and humans.[6] It has been suggested that the disease has an increased incidence in Appaloosas and Palominos.[7] In a more recent report of 15 affected individuals, Appaloosas were significantly more common in the study population.[8] To date, there are reports of alopecia areata in 6 Appaloosas,[3,8] 5 Quarter horses,[8,9] 2 thoroughbreds,[8,10] a Percheron,[11] Tennessee walking horse,[12] French trotter,[13] American paint horse,[8] Hanoverian,[8] Peru paso,[8] American saddlebred,[8] and a Dutch warmblood.[8] There are no sex predilections.[4,6] It is a disease of adult horses; the age of onset being 3 to 22 years.[4,5,7–10] In a study of 15 cases, the range was 3 to 15 years; median 9 years; standard deviation 3.9 years.[6]

Hair loss often occurs rapidly but onset may also be slow. Lesions are usually focal, circular and well demarcated, singular, or multifocal (**Fig. 1**).[7,8] Multifocal lesions are usually asymmetrical in distribution.[8] They may vary in size from just a few centimeters to 25 cm in diameter.[7] These lesions may become confluent or spread to involve large areas of the body, including the mane and the tail (**Figs. 2–7**). Alopecia may be limited to the mane and tail, producing focal areas of alopecia and/or short, brittle, dull hairs. Mane and tail alopecia may also predominate with more generalized involvement.[7,8] In the largest study group reported to date (15 cases), lesions were most commonly

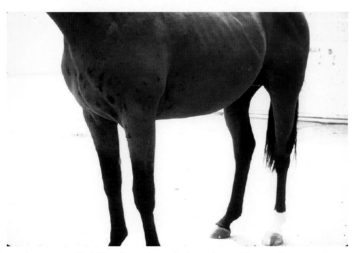

Fig. 1. Alopecia areata. Multifocal patches of alopecia and hyperpigmentation.

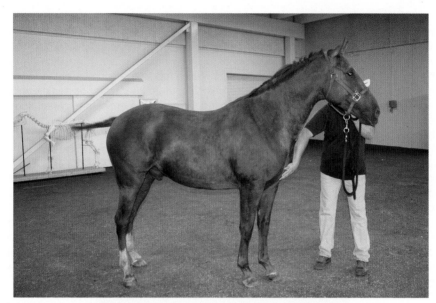

Fig. 2. Alopecia areata. Alopecia affecting much of the body, including the tail.

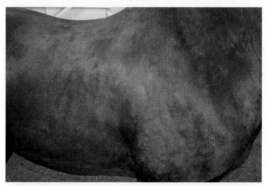

Fig. 3. Alopecia areata. Horse from **Fig. 1** showing focal to confluent patches of alopecia over the shoulder and lateral thorax.

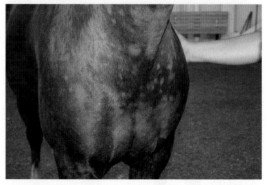

Fig. 4. Alopecia areata. Horse from **Fig. 1** showing focal to confluent areas of alopecia over the thoracic inlet and ventral neck.

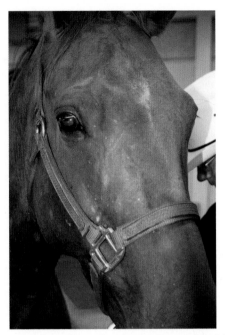

Fig. 5. Alopecia areata. Horse from **Fig. 1** showing widespread facial alopecia.

noted to affect the mane (8/15 cases; 47.1%), tail (7/15; 41/2%) and face (6/15; 40.0%) (**Fig. 8**).[8] Other areas with higher incidence include the neck and trunk.[7] In 13/15 cases, alopecia was noted to involve multiple areas of the body.[8] When alopecia has become generalized, it has often been termed alopecia universalis. This name, taken from a form of the disease seen in humans, is likely not being used correctly because, in humans, alopecia universalis is associated with complete body hair loss.[6] Affected horses have severe but not complete hair loss.[4,10,11] There is no clinically evident inflammation or pruritus. The skin in the affected areas often becomes hyperpigmented and may be mildly scaly, but is otherwise normal. In humans, nail involvement is relatively common.[6] There is a single report of alopecia universalis in which hoof involvement was also noted (onychodystrophy; ridges, laminations, splits,

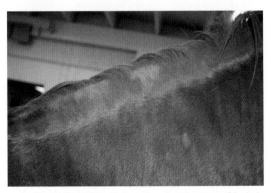

Fig. 6. Alopecia areata. Horse from **Fig. 1** showing focal areas of hair loss over the mane.

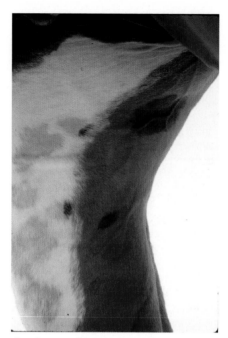

Fig. 7. Alopecia areata – focal areas of hair loss over the medial and caudal thigh of a paint horse.

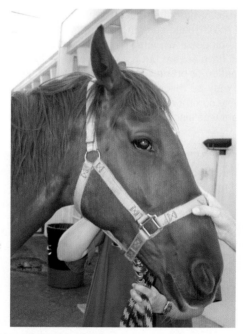

Fig. 8. Alopecia areata restricted to the face.

and fragmentation; no coronary band involvement).[13] The hoofs of the affected horse were not biopsied to confirm this diagnosis. Some cases of spotted leukotrichia with hair loss in the leukotrichic areas may be a form of alopecia areata.[5] Focal facial erythema and pruritus[14] and multifocal scales and crusts over the shoulder and back[12] have been associated with alopecia areata lesions complicated by secondary *Malassezia* sp infection.

The natural course of the disease does vary. Lesions may wax and wane in severity. In 1 study, 5 of 7 owners (71.4%) reported that the disease worsened in the spring and summer.[8] Others have mentioned improvements during the winter.[10] Lesions may go into remission within several months to 2 years. Generalized disease (alopecia universalis) usually persists,[7] but there are also reports of spontaneous remission.[9] Individuals have been noted to have recurrent disease.[3]

The primary differential diagnoses for this clinical presentation include those diseases causing folliculitis (dermatophytosis, bacterial infection) or occult sarcoid (skin in affected areas crusty, more scaly, and/or thickened). Major clinically noninflammatory differentials include anagen and telogen defluxion and follicular dysplasia.

The diagnosis is based on history, physical examination, trichography (microscopic examination of plucked hairs), and skin biopsy. Samples for both trichograms and biopsies are best taken from the margins of more recently developed, expanding lesions.[5,11] Plucked hairs that are examined microscopically may show dysplastic, exclamation point hairs that are short with frayed, fractured distal ends and shafts that undulate or taper toward the proximal (root) end.[7] Emphasis is placed on taking multiple biopsies because it may be difficult to find follicles involved in the inflammatory stages of the disease. Histologic changes seen in earlier lesions include a peribulbar accumulation of lymphocytes that has been referred to as a "swarm of bees" and lymphocytes infiltrating the hair bulb and root sheaths of especially the lower aspects of the hair follicle. Apoptotic keratinocytes, at times with attached lymphocytes, may be seen. Eosinophils are occasionally in the peribulbar infiltrate. In longer standing disease, hair follicles are in the telogen or catagen stage of the hair cycle, with variable degrees of follicular atrophy and evidence of follicular dysplasia (abnormally shaped/ distorted follicles). Pigment may be seen in the peribulbar area. There may be orphaned sebaceous and epitrichial sweat glands. Follicles may be miniaturized. There may be a mild degree of perifollicular fibrosis.[8] Because of the difficulty in finding more classically involved hair follicles, it has been suggested that clues indicating that the pathologist should cut further sections from the tissue block or request additional biopsies to find these more classic changes include (1) evidence of hair matrix damage, indicated by the presence of apoptotic cells, which may be associated with adjacent cytotoxic lymphocytes (satellitosis); (2) the presence of abnormal hair shafts in some hair follicles; (3) a subtle increase in peribulbar fibrous tissue.[5]

Alopecia areata is a cosmetic disease that does not necessarily warrant therapy and in most instances, is not treated.[8] In humans, therapies that have been used with mixed success include oral and topical glucocorticoids, the induction of contact hypersensitivity reactions in lesional areas with dinitrochlorbenzene squaric acid dibutyl ester, oral cyclosporine, and topical minoxidil.[6] In the horse, all reports of treatments and responses to treatments are anecdotal. Response to therapy is difficult to assess because of the potential for spontaneous resolution of the lesions. The author has injected intralesional steroids intradermally and observed hair regrowth at the sites of injection, although this was not intended nor observed to be a treatment for entire lesional areas. Systemic glucocorticoids seem to have variable effects. The treatment of a limited number of cases with systemic glucocorticoids has produced minimal responses.[5] There are single reports of success and failure. One horse was noted to respond to oral prednisolone and maintained in remission on 0.25 mg/kg every other day.[14] Topical triamcinolone was of no benefit in 1 horse.[15] There are anecdotal reports to suggest that twice daily topical application of a 2% minoxidil solution (Rogaine Hair Regrowth, Pharmacia and Upjohn) may be effective in the treatment of focal lesions.[15] There have also been anecdotal reports of benefits associated with the use of topical tacrolimus (0.1%; initiated twice daily). In a small number of cases, the author and others have not noted this to be of benefit (W. Rosenkrantz, personal communication, 2013).

ALTERED HAIR FOLLICLE FUNCTION
Telogen Effluvium

A stressful influence (high fever, severe illness, pregnancy, surgery, anesthesia) results in hair follicles synchronously going into the catagen and then telogen stages of the hair follicle cycle. Within 1 to 3 months after the incident, a new wave of anagen activity and hair regrowth is initiated. Older telogenized hairs are acutely shed (over days or a few weeks). Hairs can be readily epilated. Hair loss tends to be symmetric and is usually widespread (**Fig. 9**). It can be focal, then confluent, and subsequently widespread. It may also be more regionalized (eg, primarily over lateral and caudal thighs, lateral shoulders, and so forth.). The skin in the affected areas is otherwise normal. This diagnosis is usually made on a clinical basis (acute, widespread hair loss after a stressful incident). Trichography shows hairs that have a uniform shaft diameter and a slightly clubbed root end that lacks root sheaths.[16] Biopsies of the alopecic areas, at the time of alopecia development, show normal skin (anagen hair follicles). The dichotomy of alopecia and anagen follicles is explained by the fact that newly growing hairs have not yet reached the surface of the skin. Once alopecia is noted, new hair regrowth is usually visible within 3 to 6 weeks.

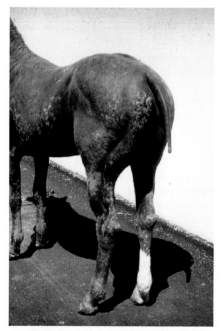

Fig. 9. Telogen effluvium. Widespread acute hair loss after a severe respiratory infection.

Anagen Effluvium

Various influences (fever, metabolic disease, infectious disease) interfere with the anagen stage of the hair follicle cycle, resulting in abnormalities of the hair follicle and hair shaft. Hair loss occurs suddenly, within days of the insult and is related to hair shaft breakage. Hair loss tends to be symmetric and can be widespread or regionalized. The skin is otherwise normal. The diagnosis is often made on a clinical basis (acute hair loss; on skin palpation, can potentially feel the stubble of the broken hairs).[16] Trichograms show dystrophic changes of the hair shafts (irregular widths of hair shaft; abnormal contours). Skin biopsies show normal skin (anagen follicles). After the insult, new hair regrowth is usually visible within 2 to 4 weeks.

Seasonal Alopecia

Seasonal hair loss to the point of developing alopecia has been noted in several scenarios.

1. Icelandic horses in Austria were noted to develop circumscribed areas of hair loss and scaling on the base of the ears, temporal canthus of the eyes, the dorsal neck, and, occasionally, the cranial shoulder. The problem developed in November and resolved in May/June, only to recur in November. Most horses were young stallions and mares. Biopsies of the alopecic areas revealed follicles in catagen and telogen and a mild nonspecific dermatitis. Feedstuffs were analyzed as normal. Feed supplements with vitamins, iodine, cobalt, and selenium prevented the problem from recurring.[17]
2. In horses from the northern hemisphere, a seasonal alopecia has been noted to begin in the spring or early summer and resolve in the fall or early winter. The symmetric alopecia is restricted to the face. The skin is otherwise normal.[16]
3. Excessive spring shedding, resulting in symmetric alopecia is noted in some otherwise normal horses, especially in the face, shoulder, and rump areas. The skin is otherwise normal. The cause of excessive hair loss is not known. Spontaneous hair regrowth is noted within 1 to 3 months.[16]
4. Some curly horses can shed excessively in the spring, resulting in patchy areas of alopecia, followed by normal regrowth. Some curly horses also experience summer shedding of mane and tail hairs to the point of alopecia, again followed by spontaneous regrowth.[18]

A treatment for seasonal hair loss has not been reported. It has been suggested that oral melatonin, which is well tolerated in horses and has been used to treat seasonal alopecia problems in the dog, may be tried (40 mg every 24 hours).[16]

Hypothyroidism

Spontaneous hypothyroidism in the horse is rare. Surgical thyroidectomy in horses has been associated with dull, rough hair coats, delayed shedding of the winter hair coat and edema of the face and distal limbs.[16,19] Alopecia was not reported. There are few reports of alopecia related to spontaneous, adult onset hypothyroidism in the literature. In 1 case, the horse had been born with a normal foal coat, but when this was shed at 4 to 6 months of age, the coat failed to regrow. At 2 years of age, a symmetric alopecia progressed to involve the entire body surface and tail; the mane and dorsal aspects of the trunk were less affected. Hairs were brittle and readily epilated. The skin was dry, scaly, thin, and easily damaged. The horse was otherwise dull, lethargic, and had low cold tolerance. There was nonpitting subcutaneous edema over the rump. The testes were hypoplastic. Skin biopsies showed dense collagen of the upper dermis and small hair follicles that contained disorganized keratinized material. The horse had a low total triiodothyronine level. Triiodothyronine therapy was given daily for 10 days. Hair regrowth was noted at 1 week after therapy, was generalized within 3 weeks, but began to fall out again 6 weeks after therapy. Reinstitution of a 7 day/mo treatment regimen resulted in regrowth and a maintenance of this coat for 4 months, after which the case was lost to follow-up.[20] In another case, the horse had been born with a normal foal coat, but at 5 months of age, patchy hair loss was noted. Hair loss was most significant over the head, neck, forelimbs, and hindquarters. Remaining hairs seemed to be the foal coat. Patches of alopecia were 1 to 5 cm in diameter. Skin in the affected areas was normal but with some hyperpigmentation. In a few areas, a few white hairs seemed to be regrowing. Biopsies from abnormal skin showed increased numbers of hair follicles and decreased numbers of sebaceous glands. Follicles contained normal hair shafts but were filled with irregular keratinized material. Total thyroxine and triiodothyronine levels were low and failed to respond appropriately to thyroid stimulating hormone. Oral L-triiodothyronine (4 mg/kg daily) for 10 days at 20-day intervals resulted in hair regrowth first seen at 10 days. The coat was nearly normal at 3 months when the horse was lost to follow-up.[21] A third reported case was an 11-year-old horse that developed symmetric alopecia over the neck, head, and flanks.[22] The diagnosis and therapy for hypothyroidism are discussed elsewhere.[16,19]

Follicular Dysplasia

Dysplastic diseases of the hair follicle are characterized by incompletely or abnormally formed hair follicles and hair shafts. The entrance to the hair follicles (follicular infundibulum) is usually dilated and filled with keratin. Follicles are usually distorted (abnormal curvatures, constrictions, dilatations). Melanin may be found in the perifollicular area. The hair loss associated with these syndromes is likely a product of both poor hair growth caused by follicular dysfunction and hair breakage caused by the dystrophic nature of the hairs produced.

Follicular dysplasia syndromes

1. Mane and tail dystrophy. Hair loss is restricted to the mane and tail. Hairs become short, brittle, and dull. This syndrome has been recognized at birth or shortly thereafter and is more common in Appaloosas and curly horses.[23] Histopathologic changes and the natural course of the disease have not been reported. Although adult onset mane and tail dystrophy has, in the past, been considered an acquired disease entity in horses (eg, Appaloosa mane and daily dystrophy[24]), it is now believed that the hair loss is related to alopecia areata.[5]
2. Black and white hair follicle dystrophy. Hair loss may be noted at birth, in juvenile or adult individuals.[24] Hair loss is restricted to either patches of white or black hair. Hairs in the affected areas are short, brittle, and dull. Diagnosis is by physical examination and biopsy. There is no treatment.
3. Curly horses are noted to have persistent alopecia of the tail (referred to as string tail or scanty tail). These horses usually also have hypotrichotic manes. These areas are characterized by dysplastic hair shafts, sebaceous gland melanosis, and follicular keratosis.[18]
4. Color dilution alopecia. A thoroughbred X Percheron gelding with a color-dilute, blue-gray coat was noted to develop alopecia at 3 years of age.[25] Hair loss started on the face and spread to the neck, shoulders, chest, and back. At the time of examination, very sparse hair was noted over the face, neck, and chest. Focal areas of alopecia ranging in size from 1 to 2 cm were widely distributed over the body.

Hair loss over the mane and tail was almost complete. Hairs were readily epilated. The underlying skin in all these areas was normal. Skin biopsies showed changes consistent with color dilution alopecia as seen in the dog (eg, Doberman Pinscher). They included the accumulation of coarse melanin aggregations in many cells of the basal layer of the epidermis, follicles that were empty or distended by keratin debris, or other follicles that were tortuous in shape and contained irregular hair shafts. Hair bulbs and perifollicular areas contained pigment clumps and perifollicular melanophages. Hair loss was gradually progressive over a 2-year follow-up. Diagnosis is by physical examination and skin biopsy. Although there is likely no therapy for this disorder, a small percentage of dogs with this disease may respond to melatonin therapy. This could be tried in the horse. See the discussion on seasonal alopecia, for a suggested equine dosage regimen.

Because of the potential hereditary basis associated with follicular dysplasia syndromes, affected individuals should not be used for breeding purposes.

Chemical Toxicoses

Selenosis

Selenium toxicosis is related to areas where soil concentrations of selenium are high or there are selenium-concentrating plants.[26] Affected individuals develop hoof abnormalities and progressive loss of the long hairs of the mane, tail, and fetlocks. Toxicoses that may produce similar signs include arsenic, mercury, and mimosine.[26] A diagnosis of selenosis is made by history, physical examination, and documenting increased selenium concentrations in tissues, soil, water, and/or feed. Therapy involves restricting exposure to selenium, oral treatment with inorganic arsenic, naphthalene, a high protein diet and/or oral DL-methionine.[26]

DEFECTS IN HAIR SHAFTS
Trichorrhexis Nodosa

Hair loss is related to weakening and breakage of hair shafts. Break points are at focal areas of swelling of the hair shafts. The swellings are often grossly visible as small white to gray nodules on the air shaft. These swellings represent frayed cortical fibers which, when looked at cytologically, look like 2 brooms pushed together.[16] The lesions have many potential causes: physical trauma (eg, excessive grooming, prolonged exposure to UV light), chemical trauma (shampoos, pesticides, alcohol, solvents). The diagnosis is made by physical examination and trichograms (cytology). Therapy is directed at eliminating the trauma.

Piedra

Piedra is a rare fungal infection restricted to focal areas of the hair shaft. It is seen most commonly in temperate and subtropical areas of the southern United States, South America, Europe, Asia, and Japan.[16] It is caused by Trichosporon beigelii. White nodules are noted on the hair shafts and represent the growth of hyphae. Hairs are weakened and break at these points. Areas affected include the mane, tail, and distal limbs. The diagnosis is based on cytology (hyphae) and fungal culture. Therapy involves shaving off the hair and the use of topical antifungals (see the article on Infectious Folliculitis and Dermatophytosis by Weese and Yu in this issue).

INFLAMMATION OF THE HAIR FOLLICLE
Alopecia Areata

See earlier discussion.

Linear alopecia

Vertically linear, often circular areas of alopecia are noted on the neck, shoulder, or lateral thorax areas.[27] There may be mild scaling or crusting. The lesions are neither painful or pruritic. Linear alopecia and linear keratosis may coexist in some horses. Although linear alopecia may be seen in many breeds, the quarter horse seems to be predisposed.[27] Although most cases are idiopathic, it is possible that some may be related to cutaneous drug reactions.[27] The alopecia is related to the development of a sterile folliculitis and possible follicular destruction. Biopsies show a lymphocytic to lymphohistiocytic mural folliculitis with multinucleated giant cells in more chronic lesional areas. Apoptotic keratinocytes and eosinophils may be found in the walls of the hair follicle. Therapies noted to slow the progression of disease include topical or systemic glucocorticoids or topical 0.1% tacrolimus.[27]

CONGENITAL ALOPECIA
Congenital Hypotrichosis

A congenital hypotrichosis was reported in an otherwise normal blue roan Percheron that was born with a partial alopecia. This progressed to being a complete, body-wide alopecia by 1 year of age. Histologic changes consisted of follicular hypoplasia and hyperkeratosis. Catagen and telogen hair follicles predominated. Excess melanin was noted within the lumina of many hair follicles and sebaceous glands.[28]

Hereditary Hypotrichosis

There are anecdotal reports of a hereditary hypotrichosis in Arabians. Hair loss is symmetric, restricted to the face, and is primarily around the eyes.[23]

SUMMARY

Noninflammatory, nonpruritic alopecias in the horse have a long list of differential diagnoses. However, the performance of a thorough history and physical examination alone often leads to an accurate presumptive diagnosis. When the diagnosis is not clear, skin biopsies can provide valuable insight. Maximal value from skin biopsies is associated with taking multiple samples. These largely cosmetic diseases are usually not associated with predictably effective therapies.

REFERENCES

1. McElwee KJ, Boggess D, Olivry T, et al. Comparison of alopecia areata in human and nonhuman mammalian species. Pathobiology 1998;66:90–107.
2. McElwee KJ, Hoffmann R. Alopecia areata – animal models. Clin Exp Dermatol 2002;27:410–7.
3. Tobin DJ, Alhaidari Z, Olivry T. Equine alopecia areata autoantibodies target multiple hair follicle antigens and may alter hair growth. A preliminary study. Exp Dermatol 1998;7:289–97.
4. Affolter VK, Cannon AG. Alopecia universalis in a horse. In: Proceedings of the 14th AAVD and ACVD Meeting. San Antonio (TX): 1998. p. 91–2.
5. Stannard AA. Alopecia in the horse – an overview. Vet Dermatol 2000;11:191–203.
6. Freyschmidt-Paul P, McElwee K, Hofmann R. Alopecia areata. In: Hertl M, editor. Autoimmune diseases of the skin. 3rd edition. New York: Springer-Verlag/Wein; 2011. p. 463–9.
7. Scott DW, Miller WH. Immune-mediated disorders. In: Equine dermatology. 2nd edition. Maryland Heights (MO): Elsevier Saunders; 2011. p. 351–5.

8. Hoolahan DE, White SD, Outerbridge CA, et al. Equine alopecia areata: a retrospective clinical descriptive study at the University of California, Davis (1980 – 2011). Vet Dermatol 2013;24:282-e64.

9. Schott H, Petersen A, Dunston R, et al. Spontaneous recovery from equine alopecia areata/universalis: case report and comparison of the disorder in other species. In: Kwochka K, Willemse T, von Tscharner C, editors. Advances in veterinary dermatology, vol. 3. Oxford (United Kingdom): Butterworth Heinemann; 1998. p. 469.

10. Colombo S, Keen JA, Brownstein DG, et al. Alopecia areata with lymphocytic mural folliculitis affecting the isthmus in a thoroughbred mare. Vet Dermatol 2004;15:260–5.

11. Middleton DJ, Church S. Alopecia universalis in a horse. Vet Dermatol 1994;5: 123–5.

12. Kim DY, Johnson PJ, Senter D. Severe bilaterally symmetrical alopecia in a horse. Vet Pathol 2011;48:1216–20.

13. Bruet V, Degorce-Rubiales F, Abadie J, et al. Severe alopecia areata and onychodystrophy on all four feet of a French trotter mare. Vet Rec 2008;162:758–60.

14. Paterson S. Identification of Malassezia from a horse's skin. Equine Vet Educ 2002;14:121–5.

15. Scott DW. Alopecia areata. In: Robinson NE, editor. Current therapy in equine medicine. 5th edition. St Louis (MO): WB Saunders; 2003. p. 215–6.

16. Scott DW, Miller WH. Endocrine, nutritional, and miscellaneous hair coat disorders. In: Equine dermatology. 2nd edition. Maryland Heights (MO): Elsevier Saunders; 2011. p. 360–77.

17. Kolm G, Zentek J. Hair follicle growth arrest in Austrian Icelandic horses. Vet Dermatol 2004;15(Suppl 1):66.

18. Scott DW. Skin of the neck, mane, and tail of the curly horse. Equine Vet Educ 2004;16:201–6.

19. Toribio RE. Disorders of the endocrine system. In: Reed SM, Bayly WM, Sellon DC, editors. Equine internal medicine. 3rd edition. St Louis (MO): Saunders/Elsevier; 2010. p. 1259.

20. Stanley O, Hillidge CJ. Alopecia associated with hypothyroidism in a horse. Equine Vet J 1982;14:165–7.

21. Hillyer MH, Taylor FG. Cutaneous manifestations of suspected hypothyroidism in a horse. Equine Vet Educ 1992;4(3):116–8.

22. Shearer D. Bilateral alopecia in a Welsh pony associated with hypothyroidism. In: Proceedings of the 5th Annual Congress of the European Society of Veterinary Dermatology held in association with the British Veterinary Dermatology Study Group, London; 1988. p. 25.

23. Scott DW, Miller WH. Congenital and hereditary skin diseases. In: Equine dermatology. 2nd edition. Maryland Heights (MO): Elsevier Saunders; 2011. p. 424–8.

24. Fadok VA. Update on four unusual equine dermatoses. Vet Clin North Am 1995; 11:105–10.

25. Henson FM, Stidworthy MF. Alopecia due to colour-dilute follicular dysplasia in a horse. Equine Vet Educ 2003;15(6):288–90.

26. Scott DW, Miller WH. Environmental skin diseases. In: Equine dermatology. 2nd edition. Maryland Heights (MO): Elsevier Saunders; 2011. p. 408–10.

27. Scott DW, Miller WH. Miscellaneous skin diseases. In: Equine dermatology. 2nd edition. Maryland Heights (MO): Elsevier Saunders; 2011. p. 448–9.

28. Valentine BA, Hedstrom OR, Miller WH Jr, et al. Congenital hypotrichosis in a Percheron draft horse. Vet Dermatol 2001;12:215.

Papillomavirus-Associated Diseases

Sheila M.F. Torres, DVM, MS, PhD*, Sandra N. Koch, DVM, MS

KEYWORDS

- Equine • Horse • Papilloma • Papillomatosis • Viral • Papillomavirus • Aural
- Imiquimod

KEY POINTS

- Papillomavirus-associated diseases in horses include classical papillomatosis, genital papillomas/papillomatosis, and aural plaques.
- Each of these diseases is associated with a different type of papillomavirus, and despite causing similar lesions, disease course and lesion distribution are distinct.
- Classical papillomatosis is usually asymptomatic and spontaneously resolves within 1 to 9 months; therefore, treatment is often not required.
- Genital papillomas/papillomatosis have not been reported to spontaneously resolve, and there is increasing evidence that genital papillomas may evolve to in situ or invasive squamous cell carcinomas.
- Routine examination of the external genitalia and regular hygiene may avoid development and progression of genital papillomas/papillomatosis.
- Horses with aural plaques may be asymptomatic or may present with signs of ear and head hypersensitivity.
- The most efficacious treatment to date for aural plaques is imiquimod 5% cream; however, this treatment option has to be carefully discussed with the owner because imiquimod causes a severe, though expected, inflammatory reaction.

INTRODUCTION

This article reviews various aspects of 3 clinical disorders associated with papillomavirus in horses commonly known as classical viral papillomatosis, genital papillomas/papillomatosis, and aural plaques. Equine sarcoids is discussed in an article elsewhere in this issue, and congenital papillomatosis is not included because to date, the various attempts to link papillomavirus with this condition have been unsuccessful.[1–3]

Department of Veterinary Clinical Sciences, College of Veterinary Medicine, Veterinary Medical Center, University of Minnesota, C339, 1352 Boyd Avenue, St. Paul, MN 55108, USA
* Corresponding author.
E-mail address: torre009@umn.edu

Vet Clin Equine 29 (2013) 643–655
http://dx.doi.org/10.1016/j.cveq.2013.08.003
0749-0739/13/$ – see front matter Published by Elsevier Inc.

vetequine.theclinics.com

ABOUT THE VIRUS
Viral Classification, Structure, and Mode of Infection

A few years ago, papillomaviruses were removed from the Papovaviridae family, where they cohabited with polyomaviruses, and relocated to their own family, the Papillomaviridae.[4] Papillomaviruses have a small (approximately 8 kb), circular, double-stranded DNA genome organized into icosahedral particles devoid of envelope.[4–6] The viral genome is composed of 3 regions: a region coding for early (E) and functional proteins (E1–E7), a region coding for late (L) capsid proteins (L1 and L2), and a region required for viral genome replication and transcription.[4,7] The L1 region is highly conserved, and has been used to identify and classify a variety of papillomaviruses strains.[4,8] The E6 and E7 proteins of human "high-risk" mucosal α-papillomaviruses (HPV-16 and HPV-18) have been demonstrated to be oncogenic through various well-established mechanisms.[8] At present, it is not known whether E6 and E7 play a role in tumor development in horses, and a recent study showed that the *Equus caballus* papillomavirus-2 (EcPV-2), commonly associated with genital papillomas and squamous cell carcinomas, does not have the retinoblastoma binding site associated with oncogenesis in the human papillomaviruses HPV-16 and HPV-18.[7,8]

Papillomaviruses characteristically penetrate squamous or mucosal epithelium via trauma, which may culminate in asymptomatic infections or during development of benign to malignant diseases.[4,6,8] Once infection occurs the virus stays latent in the basal keratinocytes, and only replicates to cause clinical disease within the differentiating cells of the stratum spinosum and granulosum, correlating with the epidermal regions where cytopathic changes and viral inclusions are found histologically.[9] Among other causes, immunosuppression and genetic and environmental factors can influence the outcome of infection.[8] In horses, smegma, poor hygiene, chronic irritation, and balanoposthitis have been suggested as promoters of genital carcinoma, and may also influence a papillomavirus infection because genital papillomas and carcinoma have been shown to coexist.[7,8,10,11] A characteristic of papillomaviruses is their high species and site specificity, with the exception of bovine papillomavirus types 1 and 2 that are typically associated with equine sarcoids.[12,13]

Experimental transmissions of cutaneous papillomatosis showed incubation periods ranging from 10 to 67 days. Disease development was unsuccessful when the inoculum was placed on intact skin but was successful when exposed to abraded skin, intradermally, or subcutaneously, supporting the need for skin-barrier breakage in order for infection to establish.[9,12]

The virus is resistant to desiccation or freezing, and can persist at room temperature in the environment for at least 3 weeks.[14,15] High temperature, detergents, and formalin can reduce the infectious capacity of the virus.[14]

Histopathologic and Electron Microscopic Findings Associated with Infection

Papillomaviruses leave characteristic footprints in the epithelium during infection. Compact orthokeratosis and parakeratosis, papillary epidermal hyperplasia with acanthosis, lack of melanin pigment, and increased mitotic index of basal cells that are swollen, have enlarged nuclei, and may form nest-like arrangements are some of the common changes seen during the growing and developing phases of viral papillomas.[5,9] In addition, large cells with pale cytoplasm, irregularly shaped nuclei, and multiple nucleoli can be seen scattered, and occasionally fused, throughout the stratum spinosum.[9] Cells in the stratum granulosum show ballooning changes and large, irregularly shaped keratohyaline granules.[9] Intranuclear basophilic viral inclusions within cytopathic cells of the outer spinous and granular layers, in addition to parakeratotic cells of the corneal layer, are identified by light microscopy and immunohistochemistry.[5,9]

Electron microscopic studies of equine viral papillomas have shown that pale cells of the stratum spinosum containing intranuclear viral particles are swollen, have large cytoplasmic vacuoles corresponding to degenerated mitochondria, and have decreased tonofibrils, with very few small membrane-coating granules in addition to large, typically irregularly shaped electron-dense inclusions.[5,9] Cells in the stratum granulosum with viral inclusions have similar abnormalities.[5,9]

Another study looked at expression of keratin intermediate filaments in the epidermis of experimentally induced equine viral papillomas in comparison with normal epidermis using 3 human cytokeratin monoclonal antibodies.[16] In advanced papillomas, the cytopathic cells in the outer stratum spinosum and granulosum did not stain with any of the tested antibodies. Moreover, in early and advanced lesions the expression of high molecular weight keratin filaments in the suprabasal keratinocytes showed an abnormal pattern that did not correspond to the normal keratinization process.[16]

A noticeable histologic abnormality of viral papillomas is the markedly reduced, or absent, melanin pigment that corresponds clinically to depigmented lesions. Hamada and Itakura[17] investigated the function and ultrastructure of melanocytes in experimentally induced equine viral papillomas. Few melanocytes from papilloma lesions were dopa-positive and, under electron microscopy, melanogenic organelles were degenerated and melanosomes were markedly decreased in size and number. Moreover, melanocytes had pleomorphic melanosomes including melanosome complexes and giant melanosomes. In advanced papillomas, keratinocytes had few stage IV melanosomes in single or cluster arrangements. The investigators concluded that these abnormalities indicate alterations in melanogenesis and melanocyte-keratinocyte interaction, and might explain the hypomelanosis seen in papillomavirus infections.[17]

Types of Papillomaviruses

In 1986, O'Banion and colleagues[18] cloned and characterized *E caballus* papillomavirus type 1 (EcPV-1); however, its complete nucleotide sequence and genomic organization was only determined 18 years later.[19] The EcPV-1 genome was shown to contain 5 E proteins (E1, E2, E4, E6, and E7) and 2 L capsid proteins (L1 and L2).[19] It was also determined that EcPV-1 is the first member of a new genus named Zeta, because its L1 open reading frame has less than 60% nucleotide sequence identity with the L1 of other papillomaviruses.[19]

The complete EcPV-2 genome was sequenced and characterized from equine genital squamous cell carcinoma and genital papilloma lesions, and genetic variants of the virus were identified.[6,7] The PV L1 open reading frame shared less than 60% (50%[7] and 54.9%[6]) identity with EcPV-1; as a result, EcPV-2 was allocated to a new papillomavirus genus named Dyoiota.[4,6,7]

A novel papillomavirus, EcPV-3, was identified and sequenced from an aural plaque lesion.[6] Comparisons of the L1 sequence of EcPV-3 with the other 2 equine papillomaviruses indicated that EcPV-3 also belongs to a different genus.[6] A phylogenetic analysis later classified EcPV-3 as a member of the Dyorho genus.[20] The genomic organization of EcPV-1, EcPV-2, and EcPV-3 is similar and contains E1, E2, E4, E6, E7, L1, and L2 proteins, in addition to a large noncoding region.[6]

Two years after the identification of EcPV-3, Taniwaki and colleagues[21] identified a new papillomavirus from aural plaques, which they named EcPV-4. The comparison of the L1 nucleotide sequence of EcPV-4 with EcPV-3 and EcPV-2 showed an identity of only 51.7% and 60.3%, respectively, suggesting that EcPV-4 belongs to a different genus.[21] A phylogenetic analysis showed that EcPV-4 clusters with EcPV-2 but not with EcPV-1 and EcPV-3.[21] A recent study coisolated EcPV-4 and EcPV-2 from depigmented genital plaques and showed that, similarly to humans, the same host can carry or be infected with more than one type of papillomavirus.[20] Pairwise alignments of the L1 nucleotide sequence showed that the EcPV-4 from depigmented genital lesions matched the EcPV-4 isolated from aural plaques and partially sequenced by Taniwaki and colleagues.[21] The investigators also described 3 other novel papillomaviruses named EcPV-5, EcPV-6, and EcPV-7.[20] EcPV-5 and EcPV-6 were isolated from aural plaques, and EcPV-7 from penile masses. Moreover, EcPV-6 and EcPV-3 were isolated from the same aural plaque lesion of a horse.[20] A phylogenetic analysis showed that EcPV-4 shared most identity with EcPV-5 (65%) and EcPV-2 (60%–62%), and EcPV-4 and EcPV-5 were considered as representing 2 novel species within the genus Dyoiota.[20] EcPV-6 and EcPV-7 shared close identity with each other (71%) and with EcPV-3 (70%), and were considered to represent the same species as EcPV-3 within the genus Dyorho.[20]

In summary, to date 7 equine papillomaviruses have been isolated from various lesions and phylogenetic analysis has allowed their characterization (**Table 1**).[4,6,7,18–21] Moreover, the presence of more than 1 virus type in the same lesion was recently reported.[20]

ABOUT THE DISEASES

As discussed earlier, recent studies have shown that equine papillomaviruses associated with classical viral papillomatosis, genital papillomas/papillomatosis, and aural plaques belong to different genera, helping explain the distinct clinical presentation of these 3 disorders, including lesion distribution and course of infection.[4,6,7] This section discusses the clinical aspects of each of these diseases.

Classical Viral Papillomatosis

Viral papillomatosis (grass warts, warts, verrucae) caused by EcPV-1 typically affect horses younger than 3 years, but no predilection of breed or gender has been reported.[14,15,22–24] It is a contagious disease, and transmission can occur via direct contact with an infected horse or indirectly through contaminated fomites.[15,24] Skin abrasion is required for infection to occur, and the incubation period of natural infections may last 60 days or longer.[15,24] Lesions start as 1-mm papules with a smooth, shiny surface and gray to white color. As the disease progresses, the lesions increase in size (0.2–2 cm in diameter) and develop a hyperkeratotic surface showing numerous frond-like projections.[23] There can be as few as 10 or as many as 100 lesions that may be arranged singly or coalesce (**Fig. 1**).

The sites most commonly affected include the muzzle and lips, although the eyelids, paragenital regions, and distal legs can also be involved.[15,22–24] Various

Table 1	
Equine papillomavirus-associated diseases, and their respective virus type and genus	
Disease[a]	**Virus Type (Genus)[Ref.]**
Classical papillomatosis	EcPV1 (Zeta)[18,19]
Genital papillomas/papillomatosis	EcPV2 (Dyoiota),[4,6,7] EcPV7 (Dyorho)[20]
Aural plaques	EcPV3 and EcPV6 (Dyorho),[6,20] EcPV4 and EcPV5 (Dyoiota)[20,21]

[a] EcPV4 was also isolated in conjunction with EcPV2 from depigmented genital plaques.[20]

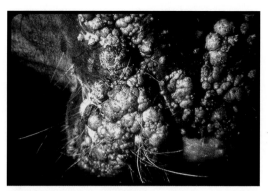

Fig. 1. Classical viral papillomatosis on the muzzle.

investigators[15,23,24] also report the genitalia as affected sites; however, investigators have been unable to amplify EcPV-1, the agent of classical viral papillomatosis, in tissues collected from genital papillomas using viral-specific primers.[3,18] This finding suggests that lesions present on the external genitalia previously reported as classical viral papillomatosis may indeed be caused by EcPV-2 or another as yet unknown papillomavirus. EcPV-4 was recently isolated in conjunction with EcPV-2 from depigmented genital plaques[20]; however, no histopathology or in situ hybridization was performed to determine whether EcPV-4 truly played a role in lesion formation.

Classical viral papillomatosis typically spontaneously resolves within 4 months, and less commonly within 9 months.[14,15,22–24] If a lesion persists longer than 10 months, an alteration of the horse's immune system should be suspected and pursued. The large majority of horses will develop complete immunity to the virus and will not become reinfected.[24]

Genital Papillomas/Papillomatosis

Equine genital papillomas/papillomatosis have been shown to be associated with EcPV-2.[7,11,25] A recent study[20] isolated a novel EcPV-7 from penile masses of a horse. However, because histopathology was not performed, the specific diagnosis and the true role of this virus in lesion formation are currently not known.

Lesions are characterized by smooth-surfaced, single or confluent grayish papules, nodules, and/or plaques (**Fig. 2**). Older lesions can evolve to produce frond-like papillomatous surfaces and keratinized horns.[13,25] Papillomas can affect multiple locations along the mucosa and skin of the external genitalia.[7,25] The lesions are more frequently seen in the free portion of the penis and glans penis in males and the vulval lips, vestibular walls, and clitoris in females.[7,13] Lesions can range from few to hundreds, in which case the term genital papillomatosis should be adopted.[25]

Genital papillomas/papillomatosis, in situ squamous cell carcinomas, and invasive squamous cell carcinomas have been considered to be different stages of papillomavirus-induced diseases.[11] The sites affected by genital papillomas/papillomatosis and squamous cell carcinomas coincide, and various recent studies have demonstrated the presence of EcPV-2 DNA and/or viral antigen in samples of genital papillomas and in situ or invasive squamous cell carcinomas, supporting the suggestion that papillomavirus induces these diseases in horses and that they represent a continuum.[7,11,13,25] EcPV-2 DNA or virus antigen has also been identified in control samples from horses with other genital lesions[7,11,26]; therefore, further studies are needed before it can be concluded with certainty that EcPV-2 causes squamous

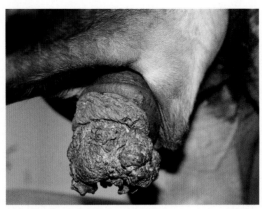

Fig. 2. Papillomatosis affecting the genitalia of a male horse. (*Courtesy of* Dr Stephen White, University of California, Davis, CA.)

cell carcinoma in horses. Recently, a horse with genital papillomatosis was followed up for 2 years during which time the lesions did not change clinically, suggesting that equine genital papillomatosis is a persistent condition that may not evolve to squamous cell carcinoma.[25]

When in situ or invasive squamous cell carcinomas develop, lesions progress to form plaques and nodules, and ulcerate. Besides the similar lesion distribution, there is an age overlap between genital papillomas and squamous cell carcinomas.[13] The mean age of horses with genital papillomas is reported to range from 16 to 18 years.[27]

Nonspecific clinical signs that horses with genital tumors may present include purulent or sanguineous discharge from the preputial orifice, altered micturition, preputial edema, inability to expose the penis, frequent protrusion of the penis, wide-based stance, and abnormal gait.[3,27] Papilloma lesions may be asymptomatic and remain unnoticed until they become extensive, underscoring the need for routine examinations of the external genitalia of horses.[27] Equine genital papilloma/papillomatosis has been suggested to be sexually transmitted, similarly to the mucosotropic papillomavirus strains (HPV-16 and HPV-18) in humans.[7]

Aural Plaques

Aural plaques (pinnal acanthosis, fungal plaque, hyperplastic aural dermatitis, ear papilloma) are well-demarcated, shiny, erythematous or depigmented lesions, typically covered with a whitish keratinous crust.[15,22,23,28] Lesions affect the concave aspect of one or both pinna, and may be single or multiple to coalescing (**Fig. 3**).[15,22,23,28] In some horses, they may cover almost the entire surface of the pinna. No predilection of sex or breed has been reported, and horses of any age can be affected; however, the disease is rarely recognized in horses younger than 1 year.[28]

Horses with aural plaques may be asymptomatic or may present with signs of ear and head hypersensitivity, such as reluctance to bridling and touching the head/ear.[22,28] Biting flies, especially black flies, may aggravate the symptoms.[15,22,28] In contrast to classical viral papillomatosis, but similar to genital papilloma/papillomatosis, aural plaques are not known to resolve spontaneously.[15,22,23,28]

The association of papillomavirus with aural plaques has been demonstrated by electron microscopy[29] and immunohistochemistry.[3,29] In 2007, Postey and colleagues[3] tried unsuccessfully to amplify EcPV-1 from aural plaques. Nevertheless, 4

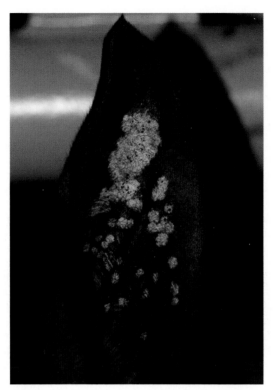

Fig. 3. Coalescing aural plaques in the concave aspect of the pinna.

novel papillomaviruses (EcPV-3, EcPV-4, EcPV-5, and EcPV-6) were recently ampli-
fied from samples taken from aural plaques,[6,20,21] and genetic and phylogenetic ana-
lyses have classified these viruses in the genus Dyoiota (EcPV-4 and EcPV-5) and
Dyorho (EcPV-3 and EcPV-6).[20]

DIAGNOSIS

Diagnosis of each of the 3 papillomavirus-induced disorders described here is typically based on the clinical appearance of the lesions, as they have fairly characteristic features. Histopathology may be required in some cases to rule out other
disorders such as verrucous sarcoid, or to confirm the presence of in situ or invasive squamous cell carcinoma in cases of genital papilloma/papillomatosis. The
previous section describes the histopathologic features of a papillomavirus infection in detail.

Various methods can be used when virus demonstration is desired. Electron microscopy will show viral particles in infected tissues, but can be expensive and is currently
limited to a few academic institutions.[9,16,17,29] The complete sequence of the 7 EcPV
genomes allowed the development of specific diagnostic probes to detect papillomavirus in classical viral papillomatosis, genital papilloma/papillomatosis, and aural
plaques.[6,7,18–21] Immunohistochemistry and in situ hybridization can identify the presence of viral protein within the nucleus of epithelial cells of infected tissues, whereas
the polymerase chain reaction can amplify virus DNA. A detailed description of these
methods is not included in this article but can be found elsewhere.[6,7,18–21]

TREATMENT

Most treatment modalities discussed here are available in textbooks, and efficacy has not been substantiated through controlled trials. Although treatment options for classical viral papillomatosis, genital papilloma/papillomatosis, and aural plaques may overlap, they are discussed separately because their course and outcome may differ, thus requiring some specific recommendations.

Classical Viral Papillomatosis

Viral papillomatosis typically spontaneously resolves within 1 to 9 months and, as it is generally asymptomatic, treatment is usually not necessary. Horses with persistent lesions should be investigated for causes of immunosuppression. In cases where papillomas become secondarily infected, are localized to areas that interfere with eating (eg, lip margin) or tacking, and are aesthetically unattractive (which can be important for shows or sales), treatment is desirable. However, the common spontaneous regression of viral papillomas makes difficult the interpretation of treatment efficacy.

Surgical excision of all lesions is curative when papillomas are single or very few. Surgical removal of a few papillomas has been suggested to induce the regression of the remaining lesions; however, Sundberg and colleagues[30] questioned this theory, and found that lesions persisted in 7 of 9 ponies treated with this modality and became more numerous in 3 animals. Cryosurgery and radiofrequency hyperthermia are other options when treatment is required.[15,22]

Various topical caustic compounds can be also tried, but because they induce an inflammatory reaction the adjacent nonaffected skin should be protected with petrolatum.[15] The most commonly used products include podophyllin (50% podophyllin, 20% podophyllin in 95% ethyl alcohol); salicylic acid (25% salicylic acid with crude castor oil, 25% salicylic acid with 2% podophyllin and dimethyl sulfoxide); trifluoroacetic acid mixture (25 g anhydrous trifluoroacetic acid, 3 g water, and 20 g glacial acetic acid); and tincture of benzoin.[15,23] The recommendation is to apply these products once daily to once every 4 days until remission is achieved.[15,23]

Intravenous or intralesional administration of *Propionibacterium acnes*, and intralesional administration of bacillus Calmette-Guérin (BCG), cisplatin, or interleukin-2 has been anecdotally advocated as immunostimulatory, and can be considered in cases of persistent papillomatosis.[15,24]

Another immunomodulatory treatment that should be considered, based on its antiviral and antitumor effect, is imiquimod 5% cream. As for most treatment modalities mentioned here, to date there have been no clinical trials evaluating its efficacy for classical viral papillomatosis in horses; nevertheless, the treatment regimen recommended for aural plaques (see later discussion) can be extrapolated for this condition. The efficacy of autogenous vaccines is questionable, and 3 to 4 treatments are required at weekly intervals.[15,22]

To reduce the chances of contagion, various management practices should be adopted. Affected horses should be isolated, and immunologically susceptible horses should not be exposed to infected premises. Contaminated water containers, feed troughs, grooming equipment, stalls, and other gear should be meticulously disinfected using formaldehyde, lye, or povidone-iodine compounds.[23,24] Fly-control measures may also help prevent disease transmission.[24]

Genital Papilloma/Papillomatosis

Equine genital papillomas have not been reported to spontaneously resolve; in fact, there is increasing evidence that they evolve to in situ or invasive squamous cell carcinomas.[7,11,13,25] As already mentioned, genital papillomas affecting the penis may be asymptomatic and stay unnoticed until they progress. It is therefore important to routinely examine the external genitalia for the presence of papillomas and to institute treatment early to avoid progression to papillomatosis or squamous cell carcinoma. Moreover, regular genital sanitation may prevent disease development, because poor hygiene has been suggested as a promoter of genital carcinoma and may also influence a papillomavirus infection.

Various topical agents used for classical viral papillomatosis can be tried for genital papillomas; however, at present there is no scientific evidence that they will be efficacious, and caution should be exercised to avoid unwanted inflammation of adjacent nonaffected tissues.

Once papillomas have evolved to squamous cell carcinomas, aggressive treatment should be instituted.[10] van den Top and colleagues[10] reported in detail various treatment options for penile tumors in horses, and commented that there is no information on randomized trials currently available to help the clinician decide on the most appropriate treatment for the patient. The ideal treatment would cure the tumor in addition to preserving the function of external genitalia. Treatment options may include surgical intervention (eg, local excision, segmental posthioplasty, partial phallectomy, partial phallectomy and sheath ablation, en bloc penile and preputial resection with penile retroversion), hyperthermia, cryosurgery (early-stage tumors or small lesions), radiotherapy, and/or chemotherapy (5-fluorouracil or intratumor cisplatin for small lesions or in combination with surgery, piroxicam, and doxorubicin).[10,13,31–34] Treatment is most successful when instituted early in the disease course, and choice should be based on the tumor size and location as well as the presence of metastasis.

Aural Plaques

Aural plaques are typically asymptomatic; therefore, treatment is usually not required. However, a few anecdotal treatment modalities have been tried to manage cases whereby the horse experiences discomfort or the owner requests intervention. Corticosteroids and antibiotic ointments have shown little to no improvement.[35] The response to various concentrations of topical tretinoin (Retin-A 0.025%, 0.05%, 0.1% cream; 0.01%, 0.025% gel) has been variable.[28] Eastern blood root in zinc chloride has been reported as a treatment option, but its efficacy is currently unknown.[28]

A recent open-label trial showed that topical application of imiquimod 5% cream is very effective in the treatment of aural plaques.[28] The 16 horses enrolled in the study received treatment 3 times per week (nonconsecutive days) on alternate weeks, and complete resolution of lesions was noted after 1.5 to 8 months of treatment. Owners were instructed to apply a thin layer of the cream to affected areas and to gently remove the tightly adhered crust that formed after treatment using a gauze sponge soaked in water. Slower response to treatment was noted when owners were not able to thoroughly remove the crusts before each treatment or had difficulties applying the cream. Most horses (10 of 16) needed sedation before each treatment, reflecting the discomfort experienced by the horses during treatment. Side effects associated with treatment included erythema, edema, erosion, ulceration, exudation, and crust formation (**Fig. 4**). These side effects were expected, and related to the inflammatory and immunomodulatory effects of imiquimod. Alopecia and depigmentation were also noted after treatment; however, the hair completely regrew in all horses 12 to 22 months after remission, and 4 of 16 horses had persistent but very small areas of depigmentation.[28] Application of imiquimod twice weekly, every other week, has also been shown by these investigators to be very efficacious, and has the advantage of less severe side effects and reduced episodes of sedation or physical restraint.[28]

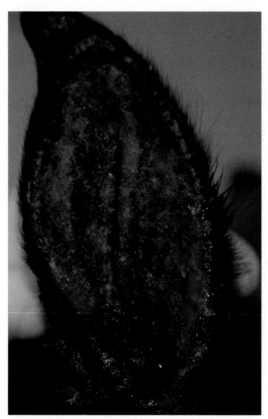

Fig. 4. Cutaneous reaction to imiquimod 5% cream on the pinna, characterized by erythema, erosions, exudation, and crusting.

One of the arguments to not treat aural plaques is the potential for horses to become head shy after treatment. However, in the study by Torres and colleagues,[28] the owners of all 16 horses that completed the study reported decreased sensitivity to touching the head and ear in addition to easier bridling.

As a result of the severe inflammation and discomfort associated with imiquimod treatment, requiring patient sedation in most cases, this treatment modality should only be considered when owners report ear sensitivity interfering with the horse usage (eg, bridling). In addition, the severe side effects induced by imiquimod have to be carefully discussed with the owner before initiating treatment.

Recently, systemic and topical antiviral medications have been studied in horses. Use of 5% acyclovir (Zovirax) has shown promise in the treatment of equine sarcoids with 32 of 47 sarcoids (68%) resulting in long-term remission with daily applications.[36]

Successful treatment of aural plaques has also been achieved without the inflammatory response noted with imiquimod (Dr Anthony Yu, personal communication, July 2013). Antiviral medications thus may serve as another route of treatment for E caballus papillomavirus infection in horses but requires further randomized placebo controlled studies.

Fly control is an important part of the treatment regimen because flies have been incriminated to worsen the lesions and to mechanically transmit the papillomavirus.

SUMMARY

Papillomavirus-associated diseases in horses include classical papillomatosis (EcPV-1), genital papillomas/papillomatosis (EcPV-2 and possibly EcPV7) and aural plaques (EcPV-3, -4, -5, and -6). Despite the similarity in lesions, the disease course and lesion distribution vary in these diseases. Diagnosis is typically based on the characteristic clinical signs; however, histopathology and/or virus demonstration may be required or desired in some cases. Classical papillomatosis typically affects horses younger than 3 years, and presents as varied numbers of gray to white papules or nodules most commonly localized to the muzzle and lips. It is generally asymptomatic, and most cases spontaneously resolve within few months; therefore, treatment is often unnecessary. Genital papillomas/papillomatosis usually affect horses 16 to 18 years old, and few to hundreds of lesions develop on the external genitalia of males and females. In contrast to classical papillomas, this disease has not been reported to spontaneously resolve and actually may evolve to in situ or invasive squamous cell carcinomas. Routine examination of the external genitalia and regular genital sanitation may avoid the development and progression of disease. Aural plaques are present on the concave aspect of one or both pinna, mostly affect horses older than 1 year, and have not been reported to spontaneously resolve. Horses with aural plaques may be asymptomatic or may present with signs of ear and head hypersensitivity. Imiquimod 5% cream, a potent antiviral and antitumor drug, has been shown to be efficacious in resolving aural plaques; however, this treatment option has to be carefully discussed with the owner, as imiquimod causes a severe inflammatory reaction requiring most horses to be sedated before each treatment.

REFERENCES

1. Junge RE, Sundberg JP, Lancaster WD. Papillomas and squamous cell carcinomas of horses. J Am Vet Med Assoc 1984;185(6):656–9.
2. White KS, Fuji RN, Valentine BA, et al. Equine congenital papilloma: pathological findings and results of papillomavirus immunohistochemistry in five horses. Vet Dermatol 2004;15(4):240–4.
3. Postey RC, Appleyard GD, Kidney BA. Evaluation of equine papillomas, aural plaques, and sarcoids for the presence of equine papillomavirus DNA and papillomavirus antigen. Can J Vet Res 2007;71(1):28–33.
4. Bernard H, Burk RD, Chen Z, et al. Classification of papillomaviruses (PVs) based on 189 PV types and proposal of taxonomic amendments. Virology 2010;401(1): 70–9.
5. Fulton RE, Doane FW, Macpherson LW. The fine structure of equine papillomas and the equine papilloma virus. J Ultrastruct Res 1970;30(3):328–43.
6. Lange CE, Tobler K, Ackermann M, et al. Identification of two novel equine papillomavirus sequences suggests three genera in one cluster. Vet Microbiol 2011; 149(1–2):85–90.
7. Scase T, Brandt S, Kainzbauer C, et al. Equus caballus papillomavirus-2 (EcPV-2): an infectious cause for equine genital cancer? Equine Vet J 2010; 42(8):738–45.
8. Munday JS, Kiupel M. Papillomavirus-associated cutaneous neoplasia in mammals. Vet Pathol 2010;47(2):254–64.
9. Hamada M, Oyamada T, Yoshikawa H, et al. Histopathological development of equine cutaneous papillomas. J Comp Pathol 1990;102(4):393–403.

10. van den Top JG, Ensink JM, Grone A, et al. Penile and preputial tumours in the horse: literature review and proposal of a standardized approach. Equine Vet J 2010;42(8):746–57.

11. Lange CE, Tobler K, Lehner A, et al. EcPV2 DNA in equine papillomas and in situ and invasive squamous cell carcinomas supports papillomavirus etiology. Vet Pathol 2012. http://dx.doi.org/10.1177/0300985812463403.

12. Cook RH, Olson C. Experimental transmission of cutaneous papilloma of the horse. Am J Pathol 1951;27(6):1087–97.

13. Smith MA, Levine DG, Getman LM, et al. Vulvar squamous cell carcinoma in situ within viral papillomas in an aged Quarter Horse mare. Equine Vet Educ 2009; 21(1):11–6.

14. Jackson HA. Papillomatosis (warts). In: Robinson NE, editor. Current therapy in equine medicine. Philadelphia: WB Saunders; 2003. p. 212.

15. Williams MA. Papillomatosis: warts and aural plaques. In: Robinson NE, editor. Current therapy in equine medicine. Philadelphia: WB Saunders; 1997. p. 389.

16. Hamada M, Oyamada T, Yoshikawa H, et al. Keratin expression in equine normal epidermis and cutaneous papillomas using monoclonal antibodies. J Comp Pathol 1990;102(4):405–20.

17. Hamada M, Itakura C. Ultrastructural morphology of hypomelanosis in equine cutaneous papilloma. J Comp Pathol 1990;103(2):200–13.

18. O'Banion MK, Reichmann ME, Sundberg JP. Coning and characterization of an equine cutaneous papillomavirus. Virology 1986;152(1):100–9.

19. Ghim SJ, Rector A, Delius H, et al. Equine papillomavirus type 1: complete nucleotide sequence and characterization of recombinant virus-like particles composed of EcPV-1 L1 major capsid protein. Biochem Biophys Res Commun 2004;324(3):1108–15.

20. Lange CE, Vetsch E, Ackermann M, et al. Four novel papillomavirus sequences support a broad diversity among equine papillomaviruses. J Gen Virol 2013. http://dx.doi.org/10.1099/vir.0.052092-0.

21. Taniwaki SA, Magro JA, Gorino AC, et al. Phylogenetic and structural studies of a novel equine papillomavirus identified from aural plaques. Vet Microbiol 2013; 162(1):85–93.

22. Knottenbelt DC. Viral papillomatosis. In: Knottenbelt DC, editor. Pascoe's principles & practice of equine dermatology. Philadelphia: WB Saunders; 2009. p. 134.

23. Scott DW, Miller WH Jr. Cutaneous neoplasms. In: Scott DW, Miller WH Jr, editors. Equine dermatology. Philadelphia: WB Saunders; 2003. p. 700.

24. Johnson PJ. Dermatologic tumors (excluding sarcoids). In: Savage CJ, editor. Veterinary clinics of North America: equine practice. Philadelphia: WB Saunders; 1998. p. 635.

25. Knight CG, Munday JS, Rosa BV, et al. Persistent, widespread papilloma formation on the penis of a horse: a novel presentation of equine papillomavirus type 2 infection. Vet Dermatol 2011;22(6):570–4.

26. Knight CG, Munday JS, Peters J, et al. Equine penile squamous cell carcinomas are associated with the presence of equine papillomavirus type 2 DNA sequences. Vet Pathol 2011;48(6):1190–4.

27. van den Top JG, de Heer N, Klein WR, et al. Penile and preputial tumours in the horse: a retrospective study of 114 affected horses. Equine Vet J 2008;40(6): 528–32.

28. Torres SM, Malone ED, White SD, et al. The efficacy of imiquimod 5% cream (Aldara) in the treatment of aural plaque in horses: a pilot open-label clinical trial. Vet Dermatol 2010;21(5):503–9.

29. Fairley RA, Haines DM. The electron microscopic and immunohistochemical demonstration of a papillomavirus in equine aural plaques. Vet Pathol 1992; 29(1):79–81.
30. Sundberg JP, Todd KS, DiPietro JA, et al. Equine papillomatosis: is partial resection of lesions an effective treatment? Vet Med 1985;80(9):71–4.
31. Fortier LA, MacHarg MA. Topical use of 5-fluorouracil for treatment of squamous cell carcinoma of the external genitalia of horses: 11 cases (1988-1992). J Am Vet Med Assoc 1994;205(8):1183–5.
32. Stick JA. Cryosurgery. In: Auer JA, Stick JA, editors. Equine surgery. St Louis (MO): Saunders Elsevier; 2006. p. 172–6.
33. Theon AP, Pascoe JR, Galuppo LD, et al. Comparison of perioperative versus postoperative intratumoral administration of cisplatin for treatment of cutaneous sarcoids and squamous cell carcinomas in horses. J Am Vet Med Assoc 1999; 215(11):1655–60.
34. Moore AS, Beam SL, Rassnick KM, et al. Long-term control of mucocutaneous squamous cell carcinoma and metastases in a horse using piroxicam. Equine Vet J 2003;35(7):715–8.
35. Binninger CE, Piper RC. Hyperplastic dermatitis of equine ear. J Am Vet Med Assoc 1968;153(1):69–75.
36. Stadler S, Kainzbauer C, Haralambus R, et al. Successful treatment of equine sarcoids by topical aciclovir application. Vet Rec 2011;168:187.

Sarcoids

Kerstin E. Bergvall, DVM

KEYWORDS

- Equine • Sarcoid • Skin tumor • Bovine papillomavirus type 1
- Bovine papillomavirus type 2

KEY POINTS

- Sarcoids are the most common equine skin tumors worldwide.
- Sarcoid pathogenesis is multifactorial, and the tumor is associated with bovine papillomavirus types 1 and 2.
- Clinical presentation varies and includes occult, verrucous, nodular, fibroblastic, mixed, and malignant (malevolent) types. The tumor is nonmetastasizing but can become very aggressive locally. Multiple tumors are common; all clinical types can be present in the same horse.
- No treatment protocol is universally effective. The tumor has a high risk of recurrence. Recurrent and large tumors carry a worse prognosis.

INTRODUCTION

Sarcoids were reported as being the most common type of equine skin neoplasm as early as 1936 and this continues to be the case to date, on a worldwide basis.[1–4] Approximately 1% to 11.5% of all horses have sarcoids,[5,6] and this type of tumor is reported to account for up to 90% (35%–90%) of all skin neoplasms in horses.[7–14] The tumor has also been reported in other equids, including zebras, donkeys, and mules,[14–17] as well as other mammals such as giraffes and sable antelopes.[18] An incidence of 0.6 cases per 100 animal-years was reported in a population of donkeys.[15] Sarcoids are nonmetastatic, fibroblastic neoplasms that rarely regress spontaneously; they can remain static or become very aggressive locally. Although the condition is not lethal in itself, size and distribution of the tumor or tumors can severely compromise the use and value of the horse, and lead to a decision of euthanasia.

PATHOGENESIS

Equine sarcoids have a multifactorial etiology (**Box 1**). An association with infectious agents in the form of bovine papillomavirus (BPV) types 1 and 2, as well as genetic risk factors, has been documented.

The author has nothing to disclose.
Department of Veterinary Clinical Sciences, University of Agriculture, Box 7084, Uppsala 750 07, Sweden
E-mail address: Kerstin.Bergvall@slu.se

> **Box 1**
> **Pathogenesis: factors needed for sarcoid development**
>
> - Equid (horse, donkey, mule, zebra) with genetic susceptibility
> - Bovine papillomavirus (BPV) types 1 or 2
> - Delivery of BPV-1 or BPV-2 into the skin (vector, direct contact, skin lesion, skin inflammation)

Bovine Papillomavirus and Association with Sarcoid Formation

The BPV types 1 and 2 of the family Papillomaviridae have been implicated as major factors in the pathogenesis of sarcoids. Viral genomes, but not intact virions, have been consistently demonstrated in sarcoid lesions but not in other equine skin tumors or equine papillomas.[19–24] The presence of BPV DNA in sarcoids has varied between 73% and 100%, with lowest rates in studies based on formaldehyde fixed tissue stored for long periods.[21,23,25] BPV represents the only papillomavirus noted to cause infection across species. BPV has also been demonstrated to induce fibroblastic tumors in mice and malignant fibroblastic tumors in hamsters.[26,27] Papillomavirus DNA is often detected in macroscopically normal skin surrounding sarcoid lesions, and local recurrence has been correlated with DNA-positive surgical margins.[21] The levels of viral DNA were also reported to be significantly higher in and around more aggressive, rapidly growing, and multiple tumors in comparison with single or mild-type lesions.[21,22] Previously BPV was considered to reside in the dermis, but later studies have shown that the infection also involves the keratinocytes in the epidermis.[28,29]

Voss[30] was able to induce sarcoid lesions in healthy horses by inoculation of sarcoid tissue or cell-free supernatant to scarified skin. These lesions were indistinguishable from naturally occurring tumors. However, in other studies the injection of sarcoid tissue extract did not always result in tumor formation at other sites of the affected horse or on donors. In these studies, BPV-1 and BPV-2 inoculated into horse skin did cause fibroblastic proliferation, but lesions did not look like sarcoids histologically (they were lacking epidermal component and fibroblast activation at the dermoepidermal junction), and what did form spontaneously regressed, which rarely happens in naturally occurring sarcoids.[31,32] These horses with induced lesions also developed BPV antibodies, a feature not seen in horses with sarcoid tumors.

The BPV types 1 and 2 belong to the subgroup deltapapillomavirus or fibropapillomavirus, formerly called subgroup A, which has the capability to infect keratinocytes (KC) and induce proliferation of both KC and fibroblasts. Conversely, BPV of the subgroup xipapillomavirus or epitheliotropic virus, subgroup B, infects KC but can only induce proliferation of the epithelium.[33]

The genomes of all BPV are divided into early and late regions. Early regions encode 3 oncogenic proteins, E5, E6, and E7, and also nonstructural proteins. The late regions encode structural proteins L1 and L2.[34] BPV infection of equine fibroblasts appears to be mainly nonproductive with respect to producing complete viruses. If only the early genes, which encode for the oncogenic proteins in sarcoid tissue, are transcribed and the late genes are not, viral capsids are not formed. Likewise, expression for L1 was demonstrated in tissue,[35] but the expression of structural proteins or capsid formation needed for virion production was lacking.[22,35] The lack of virions in equine sarcoids has further been demonstrated when equine lesion extract was inoculated into cattle and the formation of papilloma was not induced.[32] One proposed reason for the inability to produce virions is that host-specific, well-differentiated KC constitute a required cellular environment that is necessary for expression of viral capsid proteins.[36]

However, one study was able to demonstrate that apart from BPV-1 DNA being present in all sarcoid samples tested, the detection of E5 and E7 was demonstrated in sarcoid epidermis. One lesion also had the late region L1 capsomer present in the squamous layer, indicating that the virus could be productive.[29]

It has been shown that BPV-1 genomes can transform equine fibroblasts, and that the tendency of fibroblasts to proliferate faster, survive longer, and grow independently of substrate was more pronounced with more viral E5, E6, and E7 gene expression.[37] In one study, all 23 sarcoids were positive for the presence of E5 by Western blot analysis, whereas all nonsarcoid tissues examined were negative.[38] Fibroblast transformation was further associated with E5 and E6 upregulating the expression of the mitogen-activated protein kinase (MAPK) p38 in BPV-1–expressing fibroblasts. Inhibition of p38 reduced proliferation and inhibited cellular invasiveness.[39] The oncoproteins E6 and E7 are activated via the activator protein 1, and by E5 upregulating equine matrix metalloproteinase 1, which contributes to the invasion capability of fibroblasts.[39] Furthermore, E5 was shown to be able to inhibit transcription of major histocompatibility complex (MHC)-I heavy chain and to prevent MHC-I complex from reaching the cell surface by retention in the Golgi apparatus in fetal equine fibroblasts. Thus, E5-induced downregulation of MHC-I might lead to tumor cells escaping immune responses.[40] In addition, in one study an altered DNA methylation status and redox milieu was demonstrated in BPV-1–infected fibroblasts derived from equine sarcoids. The investigators concluded that this might contribute to tumor formation.[41]

It has been proposed that BPV in equine and donkey sarcoid have genetic differences in comparison with BPV in cattle, in particular within the E5 sequence.[15,42] This aspect is potentially important in the pathogenesis of sarcoid formation. However, another report suggested that the BPV E5 sequences in sarcoids and the published BPV sequences were identical.[38] Later studies showed that BPV-1 RNA from equine sarcoids had a unique deletion within the L2 protein. For this reason, no late protein is detected and BPV does not produce infective virions in the epidermis. This finding suggested that the virus differed from BPV-1 in cattle.[43]

Bovine Papillomavirus Transmission

Sarcoids usually appear where the skin is thin or at sites of previous trauma.[11,12,22,44–46] Transmission of the virus to the skin is supposed to be via fomite, rubbing, and insect vectors. BPV-1 DNA has been detected in both biting and nonbiting flies (Musca autumnalis, Fannia carnicularis, and Stomoxys calcitrans) in the close environment of sarcoid-affected horses and donkeys. Furthermore, identical viral DNA was detected in sarcoids of animals from which these flies were collected.[45,47,48] Transmission between contact animals was suggested in a population of donkeys, but in this study, genetic factors (pedigrees were not included) might have been important.[15]

BPV DNA has been demonstrated in normal skin of sarcoid and healthy horses and also in horses with inflammatory skin conditions.[49,50] In nonsarcoid skin, the BPV DNA is found in the epidermis. In one study, more than 70% of normal skin with BPV DNA was from sarcoid-affected horses or horses living in contact with cattle. Fifty percent of healthy horses living together with sarcoid horses had BPV DNA, compared with 30% in control horses.[49] It has also been demonstrated that, in contrast to sarcoid lesions, nonsarcoid equine skin is more likely to have viral DNA in the epidermis and inflamed epidermis. The presence of BPV in inflamed skin was suggested to be a predisposing factor to the disease.[51] Brandt and colleagues[29] showed that BPV DNA was found not only in the dermis but also in the epidermis in all sarcoids examined, with more DNA copies in occult sarcoid epidermis than in the epidermis of fibroblast tumors.

One study also detected BPV DNA gene E5 in peripheral blood in sarcoid-bearing horses but not in healthy controls, suggesting a possible role for peripheral mononuclear cells as a reservoir for virus. The same group has also detected BPV DNA in lesions of hoof cancer.[52] However, Nasir and colleagues[53] were unable to detect the presence of BPV DNA in 34 diseased donkeys, and concluded that latent virus in circulating peripheral blood cells does not play a role in the pathogenesis and epidemiology of the equine sarcoid.

Genetic Factors

In addition to the viral association, genetic factors also seem to be important for the development of sarcoid lesions. In horses, a breed predilection for appaloosas, Arabians, quarter horses, and thoroughbreds has been documented, whereas standardbreds and Lippizaner horses are at a decreased risk. Mules, donkeys, and zebras also can be affected. In thoroughbreds and warmbloods, the increased risk has been associated with MHC-I A3 and W13 alleles, whereas in the standardbred and Lippizaner a decreased risk is associated with decreased W13 allele and a lack of W13, respectively. Furthermore, MHC-I A3 occurred more frequently in sarcoid-affected French horses.[54–58] In zebras, the prevalence in the Cape Mountain zebras (an inbred type of zebra, descendants from only 30 animals) is 25% to 53%, compared with 1.9% in outbred zebras.[17,59] On the other hand, a study of Swiss warmblood horses did not record a higher prevalence in offspring from stallions with known sarcoids in comparison with those with sires without a known history of sarcoids.[5]

CLINICAL PRESENTATION

Sarcoids are most commonly first noticed in horses 1 to 7 years of age.[14,60] The onset of the disease at an older age is rarely reported. In horses, there is no reported color or gender predisposition.[60] In donkeys, however, young males are reported to develop sarcoids more frequently than older males or females.[14]

The macroscopic presentation of sarcoids can be highly variable. A clinically based classification of sarcoids has been suggested by Knottenbelt,[6] which includes occult, verrucous, nodular, fibroblastic, mixed, and malignant/malevolent types of tumors. A high proportion of affected horses (14%–84%) have multiple tumors, and all types of sarcoids can be present in the same horse.[6,14] Sarcoids often develop at the site of previous trauma or where the skin is thin. Exposure to trauma can induce a worsening of the lesion and a more aggressive development of the tumor.[6,22,46,61] An early age of onset, time, and number of lesions are associated with larger tumor size.

Clinical Classification of Sarcoid Type

Occult sarcoids are focal areas with alopecia, scaling, skin thickening, hyperkeratosis, and hyperpigmentation.[6] Common locations include the neck, face, sheath, medial thigh, and shoulder. Differentials are mainly infectious folliculitis (bacterial folliculitis, dermatophytosis) and alopecia areata.

The verrucous type has a rough, alopecic, raised surface, which can be verrucous and irregular. This type is usually found on the head and neck and in the axillae and groin. The main differentials are papillomas or hamartomas.

Nodular sarcoids can be divided into types A and B whereby type A are spherical subcutaneous masses and type B have dermal involvement, which precludes the independent movement of the overlying skin. The overlying skin is often haired, but can become alopecic and ulcerated. These types are often seen in the eyelid region and groin, and on the prepuce. Differentials include infectious, reactive inflammatory lesions (eosinophilic granuloma, foreign body) or other neoplastic processes.

Fibroblastic lesions are fleshy, ulcerated masses; type 1 is pedunculated and type 2 has a broad, locally invasive base. Common locations include the axillae, groin, legs, and the periocular region. Tumors can resemble granulation tissue or infectious processes, such as habronemiasis. Another differential is squamous cell carcinoma. Nonfibroblastic tumors can become fibroblastic after being traumatized.

Mixed forms (2 or more types) of tumors are common.

Malignant/malevolent tumors are aggressive and locally invasive. These tumors extend widely into adjacent skin and subcutis, are invasive, and infiltrate lymphatic vessels.

The occult and verrucous type can remain static for years if not traumatized. Nodular tumors can also remain unchanged, although less often. Any type of sarcoid lesion can develop into an aggressive fibroblastic or malignant/malevolent tumor if traumatized.

DIAGNOSIS

Sarcoids are diagnosed based on clinical signs and histopathology, as other conditions can macroscopically be difficult to differentiate from sarcoids (**Box 2**). For example, alopecia areata, bacterial folliculitis, and dermatophytosis can mimic occult sarcoids. Moreover, all types of nodular conditions (eosinophilic granulomas, melanomas, schwannomas, and so forth) can be mistaken for nodular sarcoids. One important differential diagnosis for fibroblastic sarcoids is exuberant granulation tissue. A biopsy should include deep dermal tissue and be at least 6 mm in diameter if a biopsy punch is used to harvest the sample. For thick, crusted lesions, a biopsy punch does not always reach deep enough into the tissue to reach the tumor, therefore a double-punch technique may be used whereby deep samples are obtained by a 6-mm punch biopsy introduced into a superficial opening created by an 8-mm punch biopsy.

Before verifying the diagnosis by biopsy, serious consideration should be given to the fact that traumatized sarcoids can potentially transform into a more aggressive type of tumor. Traumatic intervention should not be performed on a presumed sarcoid unless a treatment plan has been established after the diagnosis is confirmed.

Fine-needle aspiration (FNA) for cytology is usually unrewarding and carries the same risk of exacerbating tumor growth. FNA is not recommended for the diagnosis of sarcoids.

Histopathology typically reveals fibroblast proliferation. These spindle cells are often arranged in bundles, and have oval nuclei and small nucleoli. Mitotic figures are usually present in low numbers, but this can vary. Fibroblasts and collagen fibers have a whorled, tangled, crisscross, or linear or mixed pattern. Fibroblasts at the dermoepidermal junction can be arranged perpendicular to the basement membrane (picket-fence

---

Box 2
Diagnosis of sarcoid

- Differentials depend on the type of sarcoid
- Lesions clinically compatible with sarcoid and polymerase chain reaction positive for BPV-1 or BPV-2 DNA
- Histopathology: biopsy only if there is an intention to treat, should the diagnosis be verified

pattern), but this finding is not always present. The neoplastic cells are typically present immediately beneath the basement membrane, and extend downwards. A marked hyperplastic epidermis with deep rete ridges is present in approximately half of the cases. As sarcoids can be ulcerated, granulation tissue can be present along the surface. Occult and verrucous sarcoids have areas of marked hyperplastic epidermis with orthokeratotic hyperkeratosis. From the dermal-epidermal junction, the proliferating, spindle-shaped cells form a plaque-like infiltration. Hair follicles can still be unaffected and produce hairs.[62,63]

Schwannomas (nerve sheath tumors) can histologically be difficult to distinguish from sarcoids. Differentiation can be made with the help of immunohistochemistry staining for S-100 protein: schwannomas typically express S-100, whereas sarcoids stain negatively.[64]

Yet another diagnostic option is to demonstrate the presence of BPV-1 or BPV-2 DNA by polymerase chain reaction via superficial swabs and scrapings. A positive result is highly suggestive of the diagnosis. In one study, BPV DNA was demonstrated in 88% and 93% of sarcoid lesion swabs and scrapings, respectively, whereas all control lesions were negative.[20]

TREATMENT

Sarcoids are not metastatic but often show aggressive, infiltrative growth, and are notorious for a high recurrence rate after surgery. Furthermore, recurrent lesions are more refractory to treatment and carry a poorer prognosis. Spontaneous regression is rare.[60] If a horse exhibits lesions compatible with possible sarcoids, this tumor type has to be thoroughly discussed with the owner. As no treatment protocol has been universally effective, an assurance that the lesion will stay harmless or can be successfully treated can never be made.

Benign neglect is an option, especially for static occult and verrucous lesions and small tumors located where they are not at risk of being traumatized. In a study of periocular sarcoids, 15 lesions were left untreated because of their small size or uncertain diagnosis. In all these, cases treatment was later required (from 16 weeks to 15 years).[61]

Ligation of the base of sarcoids that have a stalk has been anecdotally reported to be successful. This treatment induces ischemia and necrosis of the tumor, and can only be attempted if the neck of the tumor is thin.

Surgical Intervention

If complete surgical removal with wide margins is possible, it may be an optimal choice for therapy. The presence of BPV DNA has been demonstrated up to 16 mm outside the macroscopic lesion, and local recurrence has been correlated to DNA-positive surgical margins.[65] The probability of local recurrence after sharp surgery or carbon dioxide laser was significantly higher for large sarcoids and sarcoids that had previously failed to respond to treatment.[65]

Sharp surgery has been reported to result in 50% to 64% recurrence of the tumor within 6 months. With nontouch techniques that avoid autoinoculation and wide surgical margins, the result improved to 82% (18 of 22) complete remission without recurrence.[65] In a retrospective study of 28 periorbital verrucous and nodular sarcoids without extensive involvement of the eyelid, 23 had recurrence (82%) and 39% grew additional tumors after surgery.[61] Furthermore, recurrence was associated with a more aggressive behavior. Combination of sharp surgery and other therapy, for example, cisplatin injection, has been reported to improve success rates. In one case report, surgery was combined with photodynamic treatment in a horse with multiple lesions. Some, but not all sarcoids went into remission.[66]

Carbon dioxide laser treatment was reported by Carstanjen and colleagues[67] to result in remission without recurrence in 62% of sarcoids from 60 equids, of which 45 were horses. Follow-up was longer than 6 months. Animals with multiple sarcoids had a higher risk of recurrence. In another study, 20 of 28 sarcoids (71%) resolved after laser treatment.[65] Advantages over conventional surgery are reduced risks of postoperative swelling, pain, and hypergranulation.

Cryotherapy has achieved up to 42% to 100% success with no recurrence, with an average healing time of 2 to 4 months.[46,62] A successful outcome was obtained in 11 of 14 (79%) horses treated by cryosurgery.[65] However, when small (<2 cm^2), occult, or verrucous periocular sarcoids were treated with liquid nitrogen, 91% had aggressive, rapid-growing relapses within 12 weeks of treatment.[61] Side effects reported included posttreatment alopecia or regrowth of white hair and, if used on the face or periocular area, facial nerve paralysis and loss of the upper eyelid function. Caution is also warranted when lesions are located close to joints, as septic arthritis has been reported.

Hyperthermia through heating the sarcoid with a thermo-probe has been used alone or in combination with chemotherapy, radiotherapy, or immune modulation. Only a small number of cases resolved and stayed in remission for 6 months to 1 year. In a study of periocular sarcoids, 2 lesions were treated but neither case responded successfully.[61]

Radiotherapy, also known as interstitial brachytherapy (implants of, eg, iridium-192, cobalt-60, radium-226, radon-222, or gold-198) was effective in 50% to 100% of cases, with a low (5%) recurrence rate. By use of ionizing-radiation brachytherapy (iridium-192), 8 of 8 and 13 of 15 periocular and nonocular sarcoids, respectively, went into remission.[68,69] In another study, 66 nodular, fibroblastic, and mixed tumors were treated with brachytherapy γ-radiation with platinum-sheathed iridium. Of the 53 cases that were followed up, 98% resolved.[61]

Chemotherapy can be effective, either by intralesional injections (cisplatin powder emulsion in sesame oil or almond oil, or aqueous formulation of fluorouracil) or topical application (fluorouracil, thiouracil). Mixing cisplatin with oil increases the local concentration and prolongs the retention time of the drug, and reduces the risk of cisplatin-induced nephrotoxicity and hepatotoxicity. Cisplatin is usually recommended at a dose of 1 mg/cm^3 and is deposited intralesionally using sedation and analgesia 4 times at 2-week intervals. The treatment can be combined with debulking surgery. In a large study of 409 sarcoid lesions in horses, mules, and donkeys, 96.3% went into complete remission. Large lesions, gross postoperative residual disease, and a history of having previous treatments were negative prognostic factors. Local reactions were noticed after the third and fourth treatments in some cases.[70] In another study including 21 sarcoids, relapse-free survival rate was 92% at 1 year and 77% at 4 years.[71] Complete regression was recorded in 53%. Eighty-seven percent did not have recurrence after 12 months and another 27% decreased in size.[72] In 18 periocular, nodular, or fibroblastic sarcoids, cisplatin 1 mg/mL solution in almond oil led to resolution in 6 (33%) limited-size lesions. Injectable material was noted to ooze from the lesions after injection, indicating a risk of environmental contamination.[61] In another study, the efficacy of intralesional cisplatin in combination with intratumoral interleukin (IL)-2 led to complete regression in 53%, compared with only 14% when IL-2 was used alone.[73]

The intralesional administration of 5-fluorouracil into 13 sarcoids at the dose of 50 mg/cm^3 given every 2 weeks for up to 7 treatments resulted in complete regression in 61.5% of cases. Follow-up time was 3 years. Lesions larger than 13.5 cm^3

responded less favourably.[74] Topical 5% 5-fluorouracil was used twice daily for 5 days then once daily for 5 days, followed by 5 applications on an every-other-day schedule in 9 periocular, occult, and verrucous lesions. Six sarcoids resolved, and 3 improved but later developed into fibroblastic tumors.[61]

AW4(5)-LUDES, a combination of topical fluorouracil, thiouracil, and heavy metals, has been reported to result in 35% to 80% complete regression.[61] When used in 159 periocular small occult or verrucous sarcoids, 35% resolved. Significant scarring and a detrimental effect on eyelid function were recorded in 6 cases.[61] Because of the risk of side effects, this treatment is not recommended for periocular regions, distal limbs, and coronary bands.

With all chemotherapy protocols, consideration must be given to the risk of exposing health care personnel, owners, and others who handle the treated horses. Despite the implementation of safety precautions (eg, double gloves, mask, safety bench), surface contamination with antineoplastic drugs including 5-fluorouracil was detected in 65% to 75% of samples taken from 6 cancer treatment centers in the United States and Canada.[75] Furthermore, one study detected cytotoxic drugs (CD) or metabolites in urine samples from nurses not directly involved in drug preparation or administration.[76] Urine samples were positive for CD or drug metabolites, including platinum in 4.8% to 29% of health care personnel who were handling or administering these drugs in Italian hospitals.[77] In another study, urine samples from family members of treated patients were examined. In all samples, the antineoplastic drugs (5-fluorouracil and cyclophosphamide) or metabolites of the drugs were demonstrated. Primary DNA damage was significantly increased in leukocytes of nurses exposed to CD in comparison with controls.[78] These findings stress the importance of establishing strict safety precautions for both health care workers and owners who handle the horses.[79]

Antiviral Treatments

Acyclovir, used in human herpesvirus infections, is metabolized to the active form acyclovir triphosphate in virally infected cells. It inhibits viral DNA replication, but is not known to eradicate latent virus. Topical daily application of acyclovir 5% was used in 47 sarcoids, in a few of which after surgical debulking. Thirty-two of 47 (68%) lesions went into remission, whereas incomplete resolution was observed in the remaining 15 (32%). Tumor thickness was associated with a less favorable response.[80]

Cidofovir, used for the treatment of human cytomegalovirus and human papillomavirus, selectively inhibits viral DNA synthesis and interferes with caspase-3 activity.[81,82] Cidofovir and sucralfate gel was used topically to treat 1 occult, 1 fibroblastic, and 1 mixed fibroblastic/verrucous sarcoid. All had previously had surgery but relapsed. The occult and fibroblastic sarcoids resolved.[83]

Xanthates inhibit replication and transcription of DNA and RNA viruses. Subcutaneous injections of the xanthate tricyclodecan-9-yl-xanthogenate and potassium salt of lauric acid, given at 3-week intervals, were used to treat 15 sarcoids. In some cases the xanthate was given in combination with human tumor necrosis factor (TNF)-α. Complete resolution was recorded in more than 50% of cases at an 18-month follow-up.[25]

Immune-Modulating Treatments

Bacillus Calmette-Guérin (BCG) from *Mycobacterium bovis* is an immune modulator that stimulates host lymphocytes and natural-killer cells. With this therapy, only sarcoid cells undergo necrosis, as has been shown histologically. Inflammatory reactions to BCG frequently require nonsteroidal anti-inflammatory (eg, flunixin) and/ or corticosteroid treatment. The best results have been seen with periocular sarcoids. In one study, 18 of 27 (67%) lesions treated with BCG vaccination resolved. The recurrence rate was 16.5%.[65] In another study, 26 occult or verrucous and 283 nodular or fibroblastic periocular sarcoids received BCG treatment. Perilesional injections were not effective. Of 300 tumors treated intralesionally, 69% resolved, 25% remained unchanged, and 7% worsened. Treatment with 1.1 mg/kg flunixin and 0.2 mg/kg dexamethasone was given after the third injection to prevent anaphylaxis, a potential side effect of repeated BCG injections. With this protocol, 1 horse experienced an anaphylactic reaction.[61] BCG injections can be combined with debulking surgery.

Imiquimod is an immune-modulating agent used to treat human genital warts, actinic keratosis, and superficial basaliomas. Imiquimod has potent antiviral and antitumoral activity. It stimulates both the innate and acquired immune system via toll-like receptor 7, thereby inducing a T-helper–1 cytokine response (IL-2, IL-12, interferon [IFN]-α and -γ) as well as an increase of TNF-α, IL-1, IL-6, and IL-8. A 5% cream (Aldara) was used in one study, applied topically 3 times weekly for up to 32 weeks. Fifty-six percent of treated sarcoids went into complete remission and 20% had partial remission. Overall, 80% had a greater than 75% reduction in tumor size.[84] Side effects were pain, erythema, exudation, and erosion of the area to which Aldara was applied. In an open pilot study, 46 sarcoids were treated. Eighty-two percent went into complete remission after a mean treatment time of 3.7 months (up to 10.5 months). Three sarcoids relapsed within the follow-up time (mean 29.8 months).[85] Imiquimod was applied to healthy horse skin in 2 horses, 3 times weekly for 3 consecutive weeks. Both horses developed alopecia, pain, and thick crust formation at the application site. The lesions extended beyond the application area. Histologically the treated skin showed crusting, orthokeratotic hyperkeratosis, and epidermal hyperplasia. There was a moderate, subepidermal diffuse lymphoplasmacytic infiltration. In the deeper dermis, there was edema of the tunica adventitia and a perivascular infiltration of plasma cells.[86]

Baypamun P, an inactivated parapoxvirus used as a nonspecific immune stimulator, was shown to be ineffective in the treatment of equine sarcoids.[87]

Vaccination with chimeric virus-like particles (viral antigens BPV-1 L1-E7, without viral DNA) was well tolerated in 12 sarcoid-affected horses and led to an antibody response. This response, however, did not correlate with tumoral response to the therapy. Only 2 of 12 regressed and stayed in remission (follow-up was 63 days). Others either regressed and relapsed, regressed but developed new tumors, did not improve, or deteriorated.[88] In another study, neutralizing antibody levels remained high 2 years after the third injection. This factor could potentially be protective in horses susceptible to BPV-induced transformation of fibroblasts, based on either genetic risk factors or previous sarcoid history.[89]

A single report claimed good results using autogenous vaccine.[90] However, exacerbation or spreading of the disease has been reported after vaccination.[61] Inoculation with either sarcoid tissue or cell-free supernatant from minced tumors onto the scarified skin of sarcoid-free horses resulted in the appearance of tumors at the inoculation site. These sarcoids were morphologically indistinguishable from naturally occurring sarcoids.[30]

Miscellaneous

XXterra is an ointment containing zinc chloride and extract from bloodroot (*Sanguinaria canadensis*), which is rich in alkaloids, especially sanguinarine, chelerythrine, and protopine. XXterra has been used over many years to treat sarcoids or sarcoid-like lesions. It is claimed to be immunomodulating and cytotoxic to cancer cells. Alkaloids and zinc chloride have escharotic and caustic properties. Sanguinarine has been shown to induce apoptosis, inhibit angiogenesis, and cause cell necrosis.[91–97] In an open pilot study, XXterra was used once daily for 4 to 6 days, then every fourth day, on 16 sarcoids. The treated area was covered with a bandage when possible. Total regression was seen in 10 (62%) after a mean treatment time of 2.5 months (maximum treatment period 6 months). The mean follow-up time was 34.8 months. One sarcoid relapsed within the follow-up period.[85] XXterra was applied to healthy horse skin in 2 horses, being used once daily for 5 days followed by twice-weekly application. The total treatment time was 3 weeks. There was no cover bandage. Alopecia, crusting, oozing, and erosions were seen at the application site. Histologically the treated area showed moderate orthokeratotic hyperkeratosis and epidermal hyperplasia. In the superficial dermis, there was evidence of fibroblast proliferation and disorganization of collagen fibers. There was also a mild, diffuse infiltration of lymphocytes. A perivascular infiltration of plasma cells was seen in the deeper dermis, where collagen fibers were still organized. Adnexa were absent or sparse.[86] Destruction of tissue including nose and ear cartilage, as well as deep tissue necrosis, has anecdotally been reported to occur.

Viscum album (European mistletoe) extract was injected intralesionally into 32 clinically suspected sarcoids, 3 times weekly for 105 days, in a placebo-controlled study.[98] Lesion remission was seen in 38% of treated sarcoids, compared with 13% in the placebo (NaCl) treatment group. European mistletoe contains triterpene, which has been shown to induce apoptosis in cancer cell lines in vitro. It also contains viscotoxins, alkaloids, and mistletoe lectin (ML-1), which have cytotoxic and immune-stimulating properties.

In conclusion, conflicting data exist regarding the efficacy of most of these cancer treatments, with many of the early publications being inconclusive for reasons of study bias.[99]

Factors indicating a less favorable prognosis

- Trauma to the tumor without treatment initiation
- Large tumor size
- Lack of response to, or relapse after, previous treatment intervention
- Viral DNA in surgical margins
- Treatment termination before eradication of tumor tissue

REFERENCES

1. Jackson C. The incidence and pathology of tumours of domesticated animals in South Africa. Onderstepoort J Vet Sci Animal Indust 1936;6:378–85.
2. Pascoe RR, Summers PM. Clinical survey of tumours and tumour-like lesions in horses in south east Queensland. Equine Vet J 1981;13(4):235–9.
3. Ragland KW, Keown GF. Equine sarcoid. Equine Vet J 1970;2:2–11.
4. Shaffer PA, Wobeser B, Martin LE, et al. Cutaneous neoplastic lesions of equids in the central United States and Canada: 3,351 biopsy specimens from 3,272 equids (2000-2010). J Am Vet Med Assoc 2013;242(1):99–104.

5. Studer S, Gerber V, Straub R, et al. Prevalence of hereditary diseases in three-year-old Swiss Warmblood horses. Schweiz Arch Tierheilkd 2007;149(4): 161–71.
6. Knottenbelt DC. A suggested clinical classification of the equine sarcoid. Clin Tech Equine Pract 2005;4:278–95.
7. Buechner-Maxwell V. Skin tumors. In: Robinson NE, Sprayberry KA, editors. Current therapy in equine medicine. 6th edition. St Louis (MO): Saunders Elsevier; 2009. p. 692.
8. Meuten DJ, editor. Tumors in domestic animals. 4th edition. Ames (IA): Iowa State Press; 2002.
9. Quinn G. Skin tumours in the horse: clinical presentation and management. In Pract 2003;25:476.
10. Valentine BA. Survey of equine cutaneous neoplasia in the Pacific Northwest. J Vet Diagn Invest 2006;18(1):123–6.
11. White SD. Diseases of the skin. In: Smith BP, editor. Large animal internal medicine. 4th edition. St Louis (MO): Mosby Elsevier; 2009. p. 1306.
12. Foy JM, Rashmir-Raven AM, Brashier MK. Common equine skin tumours. Comp of Contin Vet Practice 2002;24:242–52.
13. Marti Lazary S, Antczak DF, Gerber H. Report of the first international workshop on equine sarcoid. Equine Vet J 1993;25:397–407.
14. Goodrich I, Gerber H, Marti E, et al. Equine sarcoids. Vet Clin North Am Equine Pract 1998;14:607–9.
15. Reid SW, Gettinby G, Fowler JN, et al. Epidemiological observations on sarcoids in a population of donkeys (Equus asinus). Vet Rec 1994;134(9):207–11.
16. Marais HJ, Nel P, Bertschinger HJ, et al. Prevalence and body distribution of sarcoids in South African Cape mountain zebra (Equus zebra zebra). J S Afr Vet Assoc 2007;78(3):145–8.
17. Marais HJ, Page PC. Treatment of equine sarcoid in seven Cape mountain zebra (Equus zebra zebra). J Wildl Dis 2011;47(4):917–24.
18. van Dyk E, Oosthuizen MC, Bosman AM, et al. Detection of bovine papillomavirus DNA in sarcoid-affected and healthy free-roaming zebra (Equus zebra) populations in South Africa. J Virol Methods 2009;158(1–2):141–51.
19. Angelos JA, Marti E, Lazary S, et al. Characterization of BPV-like DNA in equine sarcoids. Arch Virol 1991;119(1–2):95–109.
20. Martens A, De Moor A, Ducatelle R. PCR detection of bovine papilloma virus in superficial swabs and scrapings from equine sarcoids. Vet J 2001;161(3):224–6.
21. Martens A, De Moor A, Demeulemeester J, et al. Polymerase chain reaction analysis of the surgical margins of equine sarcoids for bovine papilloma virus DNA. Vet Surg 2001;30(5):460–7.
22. Chambers G, Ellsmore VA, O'Brien PM, et al. Association of bovine papillomavirus with the equine sarcoid. J Gen Virol 2003;84:1055–62.
23. Carr EA, Théon AP, Madewell BR, et al. Bovine papillomavirus DNA in neoplastic and non-neoplastic tissues obtained from horses with and without sarcoids in the western United States. Am J Vet Res 2001;62(5):741–4.
24. Nasir L, Campo MS. Bovine papillomaviruses: their role in the aetiology of cutaneous tumours of bovids and equids. Vet Dermatol 2008;19(5):243–54.
25. Otten N, Marti E, Söderström C, et al. Experimental treatment of equine sarcoid using a xanthate compound and recombinant human tumour necrosis factor alpha. Zentralbl Veterinarmed A 1994;41(10):757–65.
26. Boiron M, Levy JP, Thomas M, et al. Some properties of bovine papilloma virus. Nature 1964;201:423–4.

27. Haralambus R, Burgstaller J, Klukowska-Rötzler J, et al. Intralesional bovine papillomavirus DNA loads reflect severity of equine sarcoid disease. Equine Vet J 2010;42(4):327–31.

28. Bogaert L, Martens A, Kast WM, et al. Bovine papillomavirus DNA can be detected in keratinocytes of equine sarcoid tumors. Vet Microbiol 2010;146(3–4): 269–75.

29. Brandt S, Tober R, Corteggio A, et al. BPV-1 infection is not confined to the dermis but also involves the epidermis of equine sarcoids. Vet Microbiol 2011;150(1–2):35–40.

30. Voss JL. Transmission of equine sarcoid. Am J Vet Res 1969;30(2):183–91.

31. Olson C, Cook RH. Cutaneous sarcoma-like lesions of the horse caused by the agent of bovine papilloma. Proc Soc Exp Biol Med 1951;77:281.

32. Ragland WL, Spencer GR. Attempts to relate bovine papilloma virus to the cause of equine sarcoid: equidae inoculated intradermally with bovine papilloma virus. Am J Vet Res 1969;30(5):743–52.

33. Campo MS. Bovine papillomavirus: old system, new lessons?. In: Campo MS, editor. Papillomavirus research: from natural history to vaccine and beyond. Wymondham, England: Caister Academic Press; 2006.

34. Shah KV, Howley PM. Papillomaviruses. In: Fields BN, Knipe DM, Howley PM, et al, editors. Fields virology. 3rd edition. Philadelphia: Lippincott-Raven Publishers; 1996. p. 2077–101.

35. Nasir L, Reid SW. Bovine papilloma viral gene expression in equine sarcoid tumours. Virus Res 1999;61(2):171–5.

36. Yuan Z, Gallagher A, Gault EA, et al. Bovine papillomavirus infection in equine sarcoids and in bovine bladder cancers. Vet J 2007;174(3):599–604.

37. Sousa R, Dostatni N, Yaniv M. Control of papillomavirus gene expression. Biochim Biophys Acta 1990;1032(1):19–37.

38. Yuan ZQ, Gault EA, Gobeil P, et al. Establishment and characterisation of equine fibroblast cell lines transformed in vivo and in vitro by BPV-1: model systems for equine sarcoids. Virology 2008;373(2):352–61.

39. Carr EA, Théon AP, Madewell BR, et al. Expression of a transforming gene (E5) of bovine papilloma virus in sarcoids obtained from horses. Am J Vet Res 2001; 62(8):1212–7.

40. Yuan Z, Gault EA, Campo MS, et al. p38 mitogen-activated protein kinase is crucial for bovine papillomavirus type-1 transformation of equine fibroblasts. J Gen Virol 2011;92(Pt 8):1778–86.

41. Marchetti B, Gault EA, Cortese MS, et al. Bovine papillomavirus type 1 oncoprotein E5 inhibits equine MHC class I and interacts with equine MHC I heavy chain. J Gen Virol 2009;90(Pt 12):2865–70.

42. Altamura G, Strazzullo M, Corteggio A, et al. O(6)-methylguanine-DNA methyltransferase in equine sarcoids: molecular and epigenetic analysis. BMC Vet Res 2012;8:218.

43. Chambers G, Ellsmore VA, O'Brien PM, et al. Sequence variants of bovine papillomavirus E5 detected in equine sarcoids. Virus Res 2003;96(1–2): 141–5.

44. Wilson AD, Armstrong EL, Gofton RG, et al. Characterisation of early and late bovine papillomavirus protein expression in equine sarcoids. Vet Microbiol 2013;162(2–4):369–80.

45. Bogaert L, Martens A, De Baere C, et al. Detection of bovine papillomavirus DNA on the normal skin and in the habitual surroundings of horses with and without equine sarcoids. Res Vet Sci 2005;79(3):253–8.

46. Carr EA. New developments in diagnosis and treatment of equine sarcoid. In: Robinson NE, Sprayberry KA, editors. Current therapy in equine medicine. 6th edition. St Louis (MO): Saunders Elsevier; 2009. p. 698.

47. Kemp-Symonds JG. The detection and sequencing of bovine papillomavirus type 1 and 2 DNA from *Musca autumnalis* (Diptera: Muscidae) face flies infesting sarcoid-affected horses [MSc thesis]. London: Royal Veterinary College; 2000.

48. Finlay M, Yuan Z, Burden F, et al. The detection of bovine papillomavirus type 1 DNA in flies. Virus Res 2009;144(1–2):315–7.

49. Bogaert L, Martens A, Van Poucke M, et al. High prevalence of bovine papillomaviral DNA in the normal skin of equine sarcoid-affected and healthy horses. Vet Microbiol 2008;129(1–2):58–68.

50. Yuan Z, Philbey AW, Gault EA, et al. Detection of bovine papillomavirus type 1 genomes and viral gene expression in equine inflammatory skin conditions. Virus Res 2007;124(1–2):245–9.

51. Wobeser BK, Hill JE, Jackson ML, et al. Localization of bovine papillomavirus in equine sarcoids and inflammatory skin conditions of horses using laser microdissection and two forms of DNA amplification. J Vet Diagn Invest 2012;24(1): 32–41.

52. Brandt S, Schoster A, Tober R, et al. Consistent detection of bovine papillomavirus in lesions, intact skin and peripheral blood mononuclear cells of horses affected by hoof canker. Equine Vet J 2011;43(2):202–9.

53. Nasir L, McFarlane ST, Torrontegui BO, et al. Screening for bovine papillomavirus in peripheral blood cells of donkeys with and without sarcoids. Res Vet Sci 1997;63(3):289–90.

54. James VS. A familial tendency to equine sarcoids. Southwest Veterinarian 1968; 21:235–6.

55. Lazary S, Gerber H, Glatt PA, et al. Equine leukocyte antigens in sarcoid affected horses. Equine Vet J 1985;17:283–6.

56. Meredith D, Elser AH, Wolf B, et al. Equine leukocyte antigens: relationships with sarcoid tumors and laminitis in two pure breeds. Immunogenetics 1986;23(4): 221–5.

57. Angelos J, Oppenheim Y, Rebhun W, et al. Evaluation of breed as a risk factor for sarcoid and uveitis in horses. Anim Genet 1988;19(4):417–25.

58. Brostrom H, Fahlbrink E, Dubath ML, et al. Association between equine leukocyte antigens (ELA) and equine sarcoid tumours in the population of Swedish halfbreds and some of their families. Vet Immunol Immunopathol 1988;19: 215–23.

59. Nel PJ, Bertschinger H, Williams J, et al. Descriptive study of an outbreak of equine sarcoid in a population of Cape mountain zebra (*Equus zebra zebra*) in the Gariep Nature Reserve. J S Afr Vet Assoc 2006;77(4):184–90.

60. Broström H. Equine sarcoids. A clinical and epidemiological study in relation to equine leucocyte antigens (ELA). Acta Vet Scand 1995;36(2):223–36.

61. Knottenbelt DC, Kelly DF. The diagnosis and treatment of periorbital sarcoid in the horse: 445 cases 1974 to 1999. Vet Ophthalmol 2000;3:169–91.

62. Scott DW, Miller WH, editors. Equine dermatology. 2nd edition. St Louis (MO): Saunders Elsevier; 2011. p. 479.

63. Martens A, De Moor A, Demeulemeester J, et al. Histopathological characteristics of five clinical types of equine sarcoid. Res Vet Sci 2000;69(3):295–300.

64. Bogaert L, Heerden MV, Cock HE, et al. Molecular and immunohistochemical distinction of equine sarcoid from schwannoma. Vet Pathol 2011;48(3):737–41.

65. Martens A, De Moor A, Vlaminck L, et al. Evaluation of excision, cryosurgery and local BCG vaccination for treatment of equine sarcoids. Vet Rec 2001;145: 665–9.
66. Reschke C. Successful treatment of an equine sarcoid. Case report on a combined surgical and photodynamic therapy. Tierarztl Prax Ausg G Grosstiere Nutztiere 2012;40(5):309–13.
67. Carstanjen B, Jordan P, Lepage OM. Carbon dioxide laser as a surgical instrument for sarcoid therapy—a retrospective study on 60 cases. Can Vet J 1997; 38(12):773–6.
68. Théon AP, Pascoe JR. Iridium-192 interstitial brachytherapy for equine periocular tumours: treatment results and prognostic factors in 115 horses. Equine Vet J 1995;27(2):117–21.
69. Byam-Cook KL, Henson FM, Slater JD. Treatment of periocular and non-ocular sarcoids in 18 horses by interstitial brachytherapy with iridium-192. Vet Rec 2006;159(11):337–41.
70. Théon AP, Wilson WD, Magdesian KG, et al. Long-term outcome associated with intratumoral chemotherapy with cisplatin for cutaneous tumors in equidae: 573 cases (1995-2004). J Am Vet Med Assoc 2007;230(10):1506–13.
71. Théon AP, Pascoe JR, Galuppo LD, et al. Comparison of perioperative versus postoperative intratumoral administration of cisplatin for treatment of cutaneous sarcoids and squamous cell carcinomas in horses. J Am Vet Med Assoc 1999; 215(11):1655–60.
72. Théon AP, Pascoe JR, Carlson GP, et al. Intratumoral chemotherapy with cisplatin in oily emulsion in horses. J Am Vet Med Assoc 1993;202(2):261–7.
73. Spoormakers TJ, Klein WR, Jacobs JJ, et al. Comparison of the efficacy of local treatment of equine sarcoids with Il-2 or cisplatin/Il-2. Cancer Immunol Immunother 2003;52(3):179–84.
74. Stewart AA, Rush B, Davis E. The efficacy of intratumoral 5-flourouracil for the treatment of equine sarcoids. Aust Vet J 2006;84(3):101–6.
75. Connor TH, Anderson RW, Sessink PJ, et al. Surface contamination with antineoplastic agents in six cancer treatment centers in Canada and the United States. Am J Health Syst Pharm 1999;56(14):1427–32.
76. Sessink PJ, Boer KA, Scheefhals AP, et al. Occupational exposure to antineoplastic agents at several departments in a hospital. Environmental contamination and excretion of cyclophosphamide and ifosfamide in urine of exposed workers. Int Arch Occup Environ Health 1992;64(2):105–12.
77. Turci R, Sottani C, Ronchi A. Biological monitoring of hospital personnel occupationally exposed to antineoplastic agents. Toxicol Lett 2002;134(1–3):57–64.
78. Villarini M, Dominici L, Piccinini R, et al. Assessment of primary, oxidative and excision repaired DNA damage in hospital personnel handling antineoplastic drugs. Mutagenesis 2011;26(3):359–69.
79. Yuki M, Sekine S, Takase K, et al. Exposure of family members to antineoplastic drugs via excreta of treated cancer patients. J Oncol Pharm Pract 2013;19(3): 208–17.
80. Stadler S, Kainzbauer C, Haralambus R, et al. Successful treatment of equine sarcoids by topical acyclovir application. Vet Rec 2011;168(7):187.
81. Bonatti H, Aigner F, De Clercq E, et al. Local administration of cidofovir for human papilloma virus associated skin lesions in transplant recipients. Transpl Int 2007;20(3):238–46.
82. Andrei G, Snoeck R. Cidofovir activity against poxvirus infections. Viruses 2010; 2(12):2803–30.

83. Scagliarini A, Bettini G, Savini F, et al. Treatment of equine sarcoids. Vet Rec 2012;171:330.
84. Nogeira SA, Torres SM, Malone E, et al. Efficacy of imiquimod 5% cream in the treatment of equine sarcoids: a pilot study. Vet Dermatol 2006;17:259–65.
85. Pettersson C, Bergvall K, Humblot P, et al. Topical treatment of equine sarcoids: a clinical pilot study comparing Aldara and Xxterra. Vet Dermatol 2011;22:466.
86. Bergvall K, Broström H, Grandon R. Clinical and histological response to topical application of Xxterra and Aldara on healthy horse skin. Vet Dermatol 2012; 23(Suppl 1):50.
87. Studer U, Marti E, Stornetta D, et al. The therapy of equine sarcoid with a non-specific immunostimulator—the epidemiology and spontaneous regression of sarcoids. Schweiz Arch Tierheilkd 1997;139(9):385–91.
88. Mattil-Fritz S, Scharner D, Piuko K, et al. Immunotherapy of equine sarcoid: dose-escalation trial for the use of chimeric papillomavirus-like particles. J Gen Virol 2008;89(Pt1):138–47.
89. Hainisch EK, Brandt S, Shafti-Keramat S, et al. Safety and immunogenicity of BPV-1 L1 virus-like particles in a dose-escalation vaccination trial in horses. Equine Vet J 2012;44(1):107–11.
90. Kinnunen RE. Equine sarcoid tumour treated by autogenous tumour vaccine. Anticancer Res 1999;19(4C):3367–74.
91. Adhami VM, Aziz MH, Reagan-Shaw SR, et al. Sanguinarine causes cell cycle blockade and apoptosis of human prostate carcinoma cells via modulation of cyclin kinase inhibitor-cyclin-cyclin-dependent kinase machinery. Mol Cancer Ther 2004;3(8):933–40.
92. Adhami VM, Aziz MH, Mukhtar H, et al. Activation of prodeath Bcl-2 family proteins and mitochondrial apoptosis pathway by sanguinarine in immortalized human HaCaT keratinocytes. Clin Cancer Res 2003;9(8):3176–82.
93. Kaminskyy V, Lin KW, Filyak Y, et al. Differential effect of sanguinarine, chelerythrine and chelidonine on DNA damage and cell viability in primary mouse spleen cells and mouse leukemic cells. Cell Biol Int 2008;32(2):271–7.
94. Hussain AR, Al-Jomah NA, Siraj AK, et al. Sanguinarine-dependent induction of apoptosis in primary effusion lymphoma cells. Cancer Res 2007;67(8):3888–97.
95. Basini G, Bussolati S, Santini SE, et al. Sanguinarine inhibits VEGF-induced angiogenesis in a fibrin gel matrix. Biofactors 2007;29(1):11–8.
96. Basini G. The plant alkaloid sanguinarine is a potential inhibitor of follicular angiogenesis. J Reprod Dev 2007;53(3):573–9.
97. Kim S, Lee TJ, Leem J, et al. Sanguinarine-induced apoptosis: generation of ROS, down-regulation of Bcl-2, c-FLIP, and synergy with TRAIL. J Cell Biochem 2008;104(3):895–907.
98. Christen-Clottu O, Klocke P, Burger D, et al. Treatment of clinically diagnosed equine sarcoid with a mistletoe extract (*Viscum album austriacus*). J Vet Intern Med 2010;24(6):1483–9.
99. Kienle GS, Berrino F, Büssing A, et al. Mistletoe in cancer—a systematic review on controlled clinical trials. Eur J Med Res 2003;8(3):109–19.

Equine Melanocytic Tumors

Jeffrey C. Phillips, DVM, MSpVM, PhD[a],*, Luis M. Lembcke, DVM[b]

KEYWORDS

- Horse • Melanoma • Treatment • Immunotherapy • Genetics • Vaccine
- Chemotherapy

KEY POINTS

- Melanomas are among the most common skin tumors in horses (second only to sarcoids), with prevalence rates reaching as high as 80% in adult gray horses.
- The overwhelming majority of melanocytic tumors are benign at initial presentation; however, if left untreated up to two-thirds can progress to overt malignant behavior.
- Standard local treatment options can be used to treat solitary early-stage lesions but do not address the underlying risk of recurrent tumor formation or the transformation to a malignant phenotype.
- Advances have been made in elucidating the molecular link between the normal process of graying and the development of melanocytic tumors with the goal of identifying new therapeutic options for affected horses.

 Video of melanoma vaccine administration in horses accompanies this article

INTRODUCTION

Melanocytes are dendritic cells derived from neuroectodermal melanoblasts that have migrated during embryogenesis to the epidermis, dermis, and other sites (eg, eye, inner ear, meninges). Through the process of melanogenesis, these cells produce a pigment called melanin, which can be found in the skin, eyes, and hair. The color of this pigment is dark and so it absorbs UV-B light and blocks it from passing the skin layer into the hypodermis, protecting it from the harmful effects of solar radiation.[1]

Funding Sources: None.
Conflict of Interest: Dr Phillips: projects with melanoma vaccine Oncept previously funded by Merial Ltd. Dr Lembcke: projects with melanoma vaccine Oncept previously funded by Merial Ltd.
[a] College of Veterinary Medicine, Lincoln Memorial University, 6965 Cumberland Gap Parkway, Harrogate, TN 37752, USA; [b] Department of Comparative and Experimental Medicine, College of Veterinary Medicine, University of Tennessee, 2407 River Drive, Knoxville, TN 37996, USA
* Corresponding author.
E-mail address: jphill35@me.com

Melanomas are tumors that arise from the malignant transformation of normal melanocytes. The cause of melanocytic tumor development is still not completely understood; however, current data suggest that tumors develop secondary to genetic mutations in the melanin metabolism molecular pathway. These mutations may increase the activity of resident melanoblasts, leading to a relative overproduction of melanin in the dermis and ultimately the malignant transformation of these cells. Genetic mutations are most commonly inherited, and certainly related to gray coat color; however, an association between increased UV radiation exposure and tumor growth has also been suggested.[2] Melanocytic tumors have been described in various domestic animal species, including dogs, cats, cattle, sheep, alpacas, and swine, although their prevalence and economic impact appear to be the highest in the horse.[3,4]

EPIDEMIOLOGIC ASPECTS OF EQUINE MELANOCYTIC TUMORS

Melanocytic tumors have been recognized for centuries in horses and are among the most common skin tumors noted in this species, comprising between 3.8% and 15.0% of all skin tumors, second only to sarcoids.[5–8] According to some studies, the incidence of these tumors in horses in North America may be increasing in parallel with the incidence of human melanoma.[9,10] Although it has been suggested that a gender predisposition exists, this has not been established.[7,11,12] In contrast, although melanomas have been diagnosed in horses of all colors, a marked predisposition has been extensively reported in gray horses, with prevalence rates reaching as high as 80% in older animals.[7,11–14] Melanocytic tumors are seldom observed in gray horses younger than 5 years and congenital tumors are rare.[11,15] Reports of breed predilection have suggested an increased risk for Arabian, thoroughbred, Lipizzaner, Camargue, and Percheron horses, but this association may simply reflect the higher number of gray horses in these breeds.[12,16–20] Although melanomas clearly are more frequent in gray horses, they also occur in nongray horses, where they are more likely to exhibit malignant behavior.[7]

MOLECULAR GENETIC BASES OF EQUINE MELANOMA

The increased incidence of melanomas in gray horses has been linked to the graying process these horses experience at approximately 5 to 8 years of age when they start a gradual loss of follicular pigmentation while maintaining a dark skin.[21,22] This graying process is an autosomal dominant trait that is associated with an increased risk of both melanoma and vitiligo.[21–24] Studies have been undertaken to elucidate the molecular basis of the graying process and associated melanocytic tumors as a comparative model for human melanoma.[13,24,25] Recent work has identified the genetic basis for the premature graying as a 4.6-kb duplication in intron 6 of the syntaxin 17 gene (STX17), which leads to the overexpression of STX17 and the neighboring gene NR4A3.[22] This duplication also appears to contain regulatory elements that have melanocyte-specific effects; transforming a weak enhancer to a strong melanocyte-specific enhancer that encodes binding sites for the microphthalmia-associated transcription factor (MITF).[26] MITF regulates melanocyte development and these binding sites within the STX17 gene provide a plausible explanation for the melanocyte-specific effects of the Gray allele, including hair graying, melanoma susceptibility and vitiligo. Although the STX17 mutation is inherited in an autosomal dominant fashion, the risk for melanocytic tumor formation and the other traits associated with this mutation appear to be polygenic.[22,26]

Mutations in melanocortin-1 receptor (*MC1R*) signaling have also been studied to determine their role in melanocytic tumor development.[27–29] Specifically, a single nucleotide polymorphism in *MC1R* (C901T) has been linked to chestnut coat color and resultant low risk of melanocytic tumor development.[28] A loss of function mutation (ADEx2) in the agouti signaling protein (*ASIP*), a known antagonist of *MC1R*, has been linked to black coat color and an increased risk of melanoma formation.[28] In addition to the upregulation of downstream genes, such as tyrosinase, enhanced signaling through the *MC1R* pathway has also been shown to result in markedly increased expression of the *NR4A* nuclear receptor subgroup in melanocytic cells.[29] As pointed out previously, overexpression of *NR4A3* has been found in gray horse melanomas, although it has not been directly associated with the development of melanocytic tumors in humans or horses.[22,30]

The genetics underlying the malignant transformation of melanocytic tumors has also been investigated. For example, copy number expansion of the *STX17* duplication has been identified within the tumor tissue of gray horse melanoma; the authors have speculated that the increasing copy number may be associated with tumor aggressiveness.[30] The Receptor for Activated C Kinase 1 (*RACK1*), a protein that serves as an anchoring point for protein kinase C, and in this role, likely plays a vital part in cellular signaling, has also been associated with melanocytic tumor transformation. Immunofluorescence studies suggest that *RACK1* expression levels can be used to differentiate between benign and malignant melanocytic tumors.[31]

PATHOLOGY AND NATURAL BEHAVIOR

Equine melanocytic tumors have been recognized for centuries as slow-growing, low-grade neoplasms. Although most cutaneous melanomas are benign at initial presentation, if left untreated, up to two-thirds can progress to overt malignant behavior capable of extensive local invasion and widespread metastasis.[3,7,12] The most common external locations for melanocytic tumors include the perineal region, the ventral surface of the tail, the prepuce, the commissures of the lips, and the head/neck, whereas the parotid salivary gland, ears, eyelids, and limbs are less common sites (**Fig. 1**).[2,4,7,8,12,32] From these primary locations, metastasis may occur by either hematogenous or lymphatic spread to any region of the body, including lymph nodes and other cutaneous sites,[4,7,33] although there is an apparent predilection for the serosal surface of the spleen, liver, and lungs (**Fig. 2**).[10,12,32] Major blood vessels (including the aorta), and even the heart, appear to be other structures commonly associated with metastatic disease.[4,32,33] Other reported metastatic locations include the spinal cord, vertebrae, kidneys, adrenal glands, and guttural pouches.[32–36] Rarely, melanomas may occur solely in visceral locations without any noticeable external disease sites.[2]

Tumor Classifications

The term melanocytic tumors encompass all histologic and clinical variants from the benign melanocytoma (nevus) to the more anaplastic malignant variants.[3] In nongray horses, these tumors include only benign and malignant variants. In gray horses, however, there seems to be a clinical continuum between benign and malignant tumors and the "melanocytic" disease process is further extended to include hyperpigmentation and infiltration of the dermis and epidermis, resulting in plaquelike lesions rather than true masses or tumors.[12,36] Tumor histology typically reveals a mildly to moderately pleomorphic population of neoplastic melanocytes, with an epithelioid to spindle shape, euchromatic nuclei, rare binucleation, variable and often high cytoplasmic

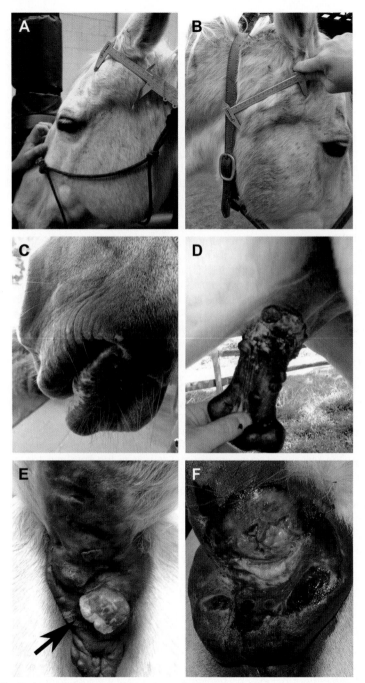

Fig. 1. Classical presentations and locations of equine melanomas. (*A*) Subcutaneous melanoma located in the temporal region. (*B*) Invasive melanoma associated with the parotid salivary gland. (*C*) Dermal melanoma located at the commissure of the lip. (*D*) Multiple dermal melanomas on the penis and prepuce. (*E*) Multiple confluent perianal melanomas (dermal melanomatosis); note areas of marked depigmentation within the tumors (*arrow*). (*F*) Large dermal melanoma at the ventral surface of the base of the tail; note further complication by ulceration and infection.

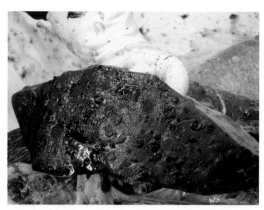

Fig. 2. Splenic parenchyma severely compromised by diffuse metastatic lesions. This image was obtained at necropsy of a gray horse that presented with a large necrotic dermal melanoma at the base of the tail. (*Courtesy of* Dr Karla Clark, Nashville, TN.)

pigmentation, and occasional mitoses.[3,37] Tumors in gray horses are classified into distinct histologic subtypes based on a combination of tumor cell morphology and location within the cutaneous adnexa. Benign-appearing collections of melanocytes located in the superficial dermis or dermo-epidermal junction are classified as melanocytomas (melanocytic nevi). Tumors located within deep dermal locations composed of well-differentiated melanocytes that exhibit dense cytoplasmic pigmentation and minimal malignant criteria are classified as dermal melanomas. Dermal melanomas are further subdivided clinically into those with few discrete nodules and those with a more disseminated variant with multiple, frequently confluent tumors (dermal melanomatosis) (see **Fig. 1**E). An alternate descriptive classification relies only on tumor cell morphology and traditional malignancy criteria to group tumors into either benign or malignant variants. Benign variants contain well-differentiated and heavily pigmented melanocytes that can exhibit a variable mitotic index and are often contained within a pseudocapsule. Malignant tumors are characterized by increased pleomorphism, variable pigmentation, moderate to high mitotic rates, evidence of vascular and/or lymphatic invasion, epidermal invasion, and indistinct tumor margins.[3,7,12]

OVERVIEW OF CLINICAL PRESENTATION

Cutaneous melanocytic tumors tend to be easily recognizable as darkly pigmented nodules; however, depigmented areas can often be identified within tumors (see **Fig. 1**E). Furthermore, amelanotic or poorly pigmented tumors may occur in both gray and nongray horses. Tumors can be localized in the deeper dermal tissues or may involve more superficial dermis and epidermal tissue. The latter will often ulcerate through the epidermis as they progressively enlarge (see **Fig. 1**F), which can also result in central portions becoming necrotic as they outgrow their blood supply.

Clinical signs in affected animals are determined by tumor location. Signs can range from simple interference with bridle and saddle caused by cutaneous lesions (which can be further complicated by ulceration and infection) (see **Fig. 1**F) to more severe signs associated with the local invasion and the compressive effects caused by internal metastatic lesions.[32] Among the latter, weight loss, constipation, impaction, and even colic associated with serious obstructive lesions in the gastrointestinal tract have been reported.[18,32] Furthermore, neurologic signs, including lameness, ataxia, and even paresis secondary to spinal cord compression by metastatic lesions, and less commonly Horner syndrome and unilateral sweating have also been reported.[32,34–36,38–40]

DIAGNOSIS AND WORKUP

The diagnosis of melanoma in equine patients is usually made on the basis of signalment (gray horse) and the physical appearance of the tumors. In select cases, including nongray horses and/or poorly pigmented tumors, biopsy can provide a definitive diagnosis. The differentiation between benign and malignant variants is typically made on the basis of all of these factors in addition to local growth pattern and the presence/absence of systemic involvement.[7,10,12,32] Molecular tests may also be useful[3,30,31,37]; however, their wide-scale reliability for differentiating benign from malignant tumors has yet to be demonstrated.

Diagnostics, such as blood work and imaging, are rarely pursued unless specific signs are present that cannot be directly accounted for by visible tumor burden, such as weight loss, chronic colic, neurologic deficits, and lameness, among others.[32,35] Blood work findings are nonspecific and may show elevated globulins, increased white cell count, thrombocytosis, or increased fibrinogen presumably attributed to the inflammatory effects of tumor burden. Diagnostic imaging can be used to determine the cause of clinical signs, although the limited number of effective treatment options for internal tumors limits their usefulness. Rectal palpation can also be useful, especially in patients with perianal melanomas, to assess the extent of these lesions and determine if they may interfere with normal defecation or could do so in the future.

TREATMENT OPTIONS

Treatment options can be divided into those therapies intended to treat the local tumor and those meant to treat and/or prevent systemic disease spread. Appropriate management of advanced cases, however, will require the combination of both approaches to achieve a successful outcome.

Local Therapies

Local therapeutic options are used to treat solitary tumors or control locoregional disease. Treatments are typically applied directly to the tumor or into the peritumoral tissue.

Surgery

Surgical resection is considered the mainstay of local therapy and is often curative, especially for small benign lesions. In some patients, however, large tumor size or anatomic location (eg, parotid region) may preclude surgery as a feasible option. Surgery can also be used to debulk more advanced tumors for palliation of symptoms and can be variably successful.[4,7,12,32,33,41]

Radiation therapy

Radiation therapy is limited in applicability because of the difficulty in treating large and/or deeply seated tumors, along with the limited availability of this modality for equine patients. Radiation, including both teletherapy and brachytherapy, has been used, however, to treat smaller tumors.[42] Teletherapy refers to treatments where radiation is supplied by an external source located some distance from the patient and requires the use of a linear accelerator or cobalt-60 unit. Horses must also be under general anesthesia during the process and the total prescribed dose is typically delivered through multiple treatments. Few reports have documented the efficacy of this type of radiotherapy in the horses because of the inherent difficulties of use in the equine patient.[42] Brachytherapy, on the other hand, refers to treatments in which the source of radiation is placed either close to or directly within the tumor tissue and the total prescribed dose is delivered in a single or small number of treatments.[42] Although both approaches have been successfully used to treat/control solitary melanomas in horses, in the authors' opinion, brachytherapy holds the most promise in the equine patient because of lower costs and ease of use. A recent advance in brachytherapy has been provided by the Axxent brachytherapy system (Xoft, Inc, San Jose, CA), which is completely electronic and allows therapeutic radiation to be delivered without the use of radioactive sources and with minimal shielding.

Intratumoral chemotherapy

Intratumoral chemotherapy involves the injection or placement of cytotoxic drugs directly into the tumor or peritumoral tissue (**Fig. 3**A). This approach has the advantage of delivering high drug concentrations to the tumor (higher than those obtained by

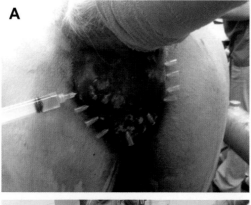

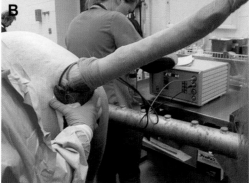

Fig. 3. Intratumoral chemotherapy and hyperthermia administration. (*A*) Large perianal melanoma that is being treated with intratumoral injections of cisplatin. Needles are preplaced evenly throughout tumor. (*B*) The tumor was then treated with local hyperthermia using a prototype microwave therapy unit (Thermofield System; Parmenides, Inc). Massive tumor shrinkage was achieved clinically in this patient.

systemic infusion of the same drug) in a cost-effective manner while avoiding systemic drug side effects. Drugs that have been used effectively in horses include carboplatin and cisplatin.[2,4,7,33,43] These can be injected directly or combined with oil (3:1 ratio) at a dosage of approximately 1 mL drug per cm^3 of tumor tissue (maximum of 100 mL of drug for the average horse). Oil emulsions are created with the goal of delaying systemic absorption; however, in the authors' experience, their main effect is transient swelling and edema of the peritumoral tissue. Response rates for equine melanomas treated with intratumoral cisplatin have been reported as high as 81%, and are suggested to be inversely related to tumor volume.[43]

Chemotherapy can also be delivered into the tumor through the use of biodegradable drug-containing beads. Such beads are marketed under the trade name Matrix III beads (Royer Biomedical, Inc, Frederick, MD) and can be impregnated with either cisplatin (1.6 mg/bead) or carboplatin (4.6 mg/bead). In one retrospective study, a variety of cutaneous tumor types, including 14 melanomas, were treated by the surgical implantation of cisplatin-containing beads. Treatment consisted of either the implantation of a single bead directly into smaller tumors or multiple beads ($\sim$2 cm apart) into the wound bed of surgically debulked larger tumors. Most horses received a single treatment and all but one remained tumor free more than 2 years after implantation.[44]

Strategies have also been developed to improve the activity of intratumoral chemotherapy for the treatment of solid tumors in horses. Drug additives, such as epinephrine or sesame oil, may be used to delay systemic absorption. Other modalities, including hyperthermia and electrochemotherapy, can also be used to increase tumor cell uptake of chemotherapy and thus improve clinical response. Hyperthermia is a therapeutic modality in which localized heat is used either alone or in combination with chemotherapy to treat solid tumors. Tumor tissue can be effectively heated using ultrasound, radiofrequency, or microwave energy.[45] Radiofrequency techniques have been described for the treatment of equine melanomas but are limited to small ($\sim$2–3 cm) and easily accessible lesions.[46] A novel system that uses microwave energy (Thermofield System, Parmenides, Inc, Franklin, TN) has also been reported and allows for the treatment of larger and more invasive tumors and is especially effective when combined with intratumoral chemotherapy.[47] In a recent preclinical study, this novel system was used to treat a series of patients, including 2 horses with locally advanced solid tumors. Complete clinical responses were achieved in both equine patients, one of which had an extremely large tail-base melanoma. These clinical results led to the development of an advanced commercial thermotherapy unit that is now available (Thermofield System, Parmenides, Inc). In the authors' experience, this combination of hyperthermia and intratumoral chemotherapy has proven quite effective for treating locoregionally advanced disease that is often resistant to treatment with chemotherapy alone (see **Fig. 3**B).

Electrochemotherapy uses controlled electrical pulses delivered directly to the tumor as a means to enhance the uptake of cytotoxic drugs by tumor cells. The electrical pulses are delivered immediately after drug injection via a set of electrodes placed directly into the tumor while the horse is under general anesthesia.[48] This modality appears to be effective for the treatment of equine sarcoids (<5 cm diameter),[48,49] but only 2 clinical reports have described its use for equine melanomas. In the first report, a relatively large buccal tumor was treated and resulted in a 50% reduction in size that was maintained for more than 1 year before being lost to follow-up.[50] The second report involved a horse with multiple melanomas that was treated with a combination of surgical resection and electrochemotherapy. Tumor control appeared to be poor, with the horse experiencing tumor progression 5 months after treatment.[51]

Intratumoral immunotherapy

Other agents that have shown activity when injected directly into equine melanomas include DNA plasmids encoding the cytokines interleukin (IL)-12 and IL-18.[52,53] These cytokines have antitumor effects through the activation of cytotoxic T cells, the production of interferon-γ, and the induction of apoptosis in tumor cells.[54] Two studies evaluated the use of these agents in tumor-bearing gray horses. The first involved the intratumoral injection of DNA plasmids encoding the human IL-12 gene in a cohort of 7 gray horses.[52] The second involved the intratumoral injection of DNA plasmids containing either equine IL-12 or IL-18 in a cohort of 26 gray horses.[53] Shrinkage of the injected tumors was observed in most horses from each study and the therapy appeared to be safe and well tolerated.[55,56] Unfortunately, these treatments are not commercially available and their benefits appear to be limited to injected lesions (ie, no systemic antitumor effects).

Miscellaneous

A variety of other agents have been anecdotally used to treat melanocytic tumors. These compounds range from topical 5-Fluorouracil (5-FU) and Imiquimod 5% (Aldara) creams to herbal compounds, such as XXterra (Larson Labs, Fort Collins, CO) based in bloodroot powder. Bacillus Calmette-Guerin intratumor injections have also been proposed; however, results for equine melanomas have been disappointing.[7] Cryotherapy can also be considered as a complementary measure to sterilize surgical wound beds or to treat small tumors. These treatments can typically be performed in standing sedated horses.[2,7,10,25,57]

Systemic Therapies

In comparison to the variety of available local treatment options for horses with melanoma, there are few effective systemic therapies available to treat/prevent disease spread. The only reported options are immunotherapeutics. These are treatments that are meant to indirectly or directly stimulate an antitumor immune response.

Nonspecific (indirect) antitumor immunotherapy

Nonspecific immunotherapies do not directly target tumor cells or tumor-related antigens; rather, they stimulate the immune system in a general way that may also result in increased activity against tumors. An example of nonspecific immunotherapy is the use of cimetidine for the treatment of horses with melanoma. Cimetidine is a well-known histamine (H2) receptor antagonist that may exert antitumor effects by several mechanisms, including the inhibition of H2 receptors on tumor cells as well as the "immune stimulatory" effects of activating natural killer cells and the blocking of H2 receptor–mediated activation of immunosuppressive regulatory T cells.[58,59] Described oral doses for horses with melanoma range from 1.6 mg/kg every 24 hours to 7.5 mg/kg twice a day or 3 times a day.[60–63] Although one small case series has described a clinical benefit in treated horses,[60] several larger clinical trials have failed to replicate these results,[61–63] and, thus, the clinical effectiveness of cimetidine "immunotherapy" remains questionable.

Specific antitumor immunotherapy

An alternate approach for systemic immunotherapy involves the direct targeting of tumor-associated antigens (TAA). These are proteins that are preferentially expressed in tumor tissue.[64] This preferential expression may occur either in a temporal or spatial fashion and allows for the targeting of tumor tissue while sparing normal tissue. An example of temporally restricted expression is a tumor that expresses an embryologic antigen in an adult animal (eg, CEA in human colon cancer). A spatially restricted protein is one in which the expression is limited to tumor tissue with minimal to no expression in other tissues. Identification of these proteins allows for the creation of immunotherapeutics or "vaccines" designed to elicit specific immune responses against cells that contain them regardless of their location within the body. The ultimate goal in creating a "cancer vaccine" is the generation of an antitumor immune response that results in clinical regression of a primary tumor and any associated metastatic lesions. There are numerous types of cancer vaccines, but only 2 have been specifically used for the treatment of equine melanoma; namely, whole-tumor cell autogenous vaccines[32,65] and a DNA-based vaccine.[66] Autogenous vaccines are created by isolating cells from the excised tumor of an individual equine patient, which are then processed in vitro into a vaccine formulation, and then readministered to the same patient. There are 2 reports describing the use of an autogenous vaccine in melanoma-bearing horses.[32,65] Tumor regressions and subjective improvement in well-being were reported in both studies. Unfortunately, the studies involved relatively small numbers of horses that were also treated with more than just the vaccine, and, thus, the true benefit of these vaccines is unknown.

DNA-based vaccines are created by first identifying an appropriate tumor-associated antigen. These antigens are tumor-specific proteins whose DNA sequence is used to create the vaccine. The DNA sequence is typically cloned into a molecular vector that allows for the in vivo expression of the encoded protein. Most molecular vectors also have immune stimulatory properties that improve the efficiency of the vaccine in generating an immune response against the expressed protein. This molecular construct (ie, DNA sequence cloned into vector) is often administered to the patient by intramuscular injection and thus resembles a "vaccination," although it may be more appropriately referred to as gene therapy. One logical tumor-associated antigen that can be targeted in melanomas via a DNA-based vaccine is the protein tyrosinase, an enzyme crucial for melanin pigment synthesis. Tyrosinase has the ideal characteristics for a tumor-associated antigen because its expression is virtually limited to melanocytes.[67] Furthermore, in melanomas (including equine variants), the tyrosinase expression appears to be constitutively increased compared with normal melanocytes.[68] A USDA-approved xenogenic DNA vaccine encoding human tyrosinase (HuTyr) is available for treatment of canine melanoma (Oncept; Merial, Ltd, Athens, GA).[69] This vaccine exploits the close homology (92%) between human and canine tyrosinase to generate a tyrosinase-specific antitumor response and dramatically improves survival in treated dogs.[70] In comparison, the equine tyrosinase sequence shares 90% homology to the human sequence; therefore, cross-reactivity of HuTyr DNA vaccine in the horse would be expected.

The use of this vaccine has been evaluated in a small cohort of normal horses (see Video 1).[66,71] The results from this report suggest the vaccine is safe and effective in generating antityrosinase-directed immune responses in horses.[66] The authors have also used this vaccine in an off-label fashion to treat a large number (>50) of tumor-bearing horses, with some exhibiting dramatic tumor shrinkage. A clinical trial was funded by the Morris Animal Foundation (D12EQ-037) to further evaluate the safety and activity of various doses of the Oncept vaccine in tumor-bearing horses (**Fig. 4**). Initial results are promising, with most horses demonstrating tumor shrinkage following vaccination. Although the vaccine is not currently labeled for use in the equine patient, these studies suggest off-label use may be beneficial in horses with melanoma.[66,68,71] Further work evaluating the role of other melanocyte-specific proteins as targets for immunotherapy is ongoing. Researchers at the University of Florida are also investigating a tumor-targeting vaccine based on the disialoganglioside GD3

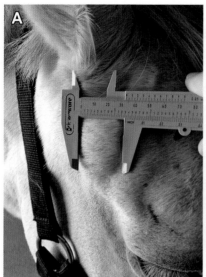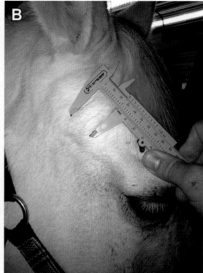

Fig. 4. Dermal melanoma being treated with the Oncept melanoma vaccine (Merial, Ltd, Athens, GA). (*A*) Tumor before treatment. (*B*) Results after treatment with 4 doses of vaccine; note reduction in tumor size and volume (tumor appears significantly flatter).

cell surface antigen to treat horses with melanoma, although no published information on the clinical activity of this vaccine is available.

PROGNOSIS AND COMPARATIVE ASPECTS

The clinical outcome in horses with melanoma(s) is mainly determined by initial tumor size and extent.[2,12] Histopathologic classification and availability of treatment options also has some impact.[3] In general, melanomas in gray horses expand slowly or may show tumor dormancy for long periods, even years. If left untreated, many will eventually acquire malignant clinical behavior with respect to both local growth and systemic spread.[7] Ultimately, the time from tumor appearance and/or diagnosis to the time that advanced locoregional or systemic disease is diagnosed will vary from animal to animal and no formal survival time studies have been performed in the horse. In both humans and dogs, malignant melanomas may result in widespread life-threatening metastases; however, unlike in humans, most horses will not die from metastatic disease but are euthanized because of local disease complications (eg, large perianal melanomas that prevent normal defecation or rupture, become ulcerated, infected, and painful). Systemic signs associated with advanced metastatic disease in both humans and horses are varied, including chronic weight loss, neurologic symptoms, and respiratory signs, among others. Some of the more common equine-specific signs associated with advanced disease include colic symptoms from gastrointestinal invasion, difficulty defecating from obstructive lesions, nasal bleeding, or neurologic signs from guttural pouch involvement. When such advanced symptoms are observed in horses, they can be difficult to treat and will commonly be the cause of death or reason for euthanasia. The development of new local and systemic therapies, including advances in accessible radiotherapy and molecularly targeted therapies, will prove useful in managing these challenging cases.

SUPPLEMENTARY DATA

Video related to this article http://dx.doi.org/10.1016/j.cveq.2013.08.008.

REFERENCES

1. Agar N, Young AR. Melanogenesis: a photoprotective response to DNA damage? Mutat Res 2005;571:121–32.
2. Buechner-Maxwell V. Skin tumors. In: Robinson NE, editor. Current therapy in equine medicine. 6th edition. St Louis (MO): Mosby; 2009. p. 692–7.
3. Smith SH, Goldschmidt MH, McManus PM. A comparative review of melanocytic neoplasms. Vet Pathol 2002;39:651–78.
4. White SD, Evans AG, VanMetre DC. Diseases of the skin, melanoma. In: Smith BP, editor. Large animal internal medicine. 4th edition. St Louis (MO): Mosby; 2009. p. 1327–31.
5. McFadyean S. Equine melanomatosis. J Comp Med 1933;46:186–204.
6. Cotchin E. Tumours in farm animals: a survey of tumours examined at the Royal Veterinary College, London, during 1950-60. Vet Rec 1960;72:816–23.
7. Johnson PJ. Dermatologic tumors (excluding sarcoids). Vet Clin North Am Equine Pract 1998;14:625–58.
8. Sundberg J, Burnstein T, Page E, et al. Neoplasms of equidae. J Am Vet Med Assoc 1977;170(2):150–2.
9. Linos E, Swetter SM, Cockburn MG, et al. Increasing burden of melanoma in the United States. J Invest Dermatol 2009;129:1666–74.
10. Goetz TE, Long MT. Treatment of melanomas in horses. Compend Contin Educ Pract Vet 1993;15:608–10.
11. Foley GL, Valentine BA, Kincaid AL. Congenital and acquired melanocytomas (benign melanomas) in eighteen young horses. Vet Pathol 1991;28:363.
12. Valentine BA. Equine melanocytic tumors: a retrospective study of 53 horses (1988–1991). J Vet Intern Med 1995;9:291–7.
13. Levene A. Equine melanotic disease. Tumori 1971;57:133–68.
14. Comfort A. Coat-colour and longevity in thoroughbred mares. Nature 1958;182:1531–2.
15. Rodríguez M, García-Barona V, Peña L, et al. Gray horse melanotic condition: a pigmentary disorder. J Equine Vet Sci 1997;17:677–81.
16. Cox JH, DeBoes RM, Leipold HW. Congenital malignant melanoma in two foals. J Am Vet Med Assoc 1989;194:945–7.
17. Mullowney PC. Dermatologic diseases of horses. Part IV. Environmental, congenital and neoplastic diseases. Compend Contin Educ Pract Vet 1985;7:S22–34.
18. Seltenhammer MH, Simhofer H, Scherzer S, et al. Equine melanoma in a population of 296 gray Lipizzaner horses. Equine Vet J 2003;35:153–7.
19. Fleury C, Bérard F, Leblond A, et al. The study of cutaneous melanomas in Camargue-type gray-skinned horses (2): epidemiological survey. Pigment Cell Res 2000;13:47–51.
20. Schaffer PA, Wobeser B, Martin LE, et al. Cutaneous neoplastic lesions of equids in the central United States and Canada: 3,351 biopsy specimens from 3,272 equids (2000-2010). J Am Vet Med Assoc 2013;242:99–104.
21. Valentine BA. Survey of equine cutaneous neoplasia in the Pacific Northwest. J Vet Diagn Invest 2006;18:123–6.
22. Rosengren PG, Golovko A, Sundström E, et al. A cis-acting regulatory mutation causes premature hair graying and susceptibility to melanoma in the horse. Nat Genet 2008;40:1004–9.

23. Curik I, Drumi T, Seltenhammer M, et al. Complex inheritance of melanoma and pigmentation of coat and skin in gray horses. PLoS Genet 2013;9:1–9.
24. Rieder S, Stricker C, Joerg H, et al. A comparative genetic approach for the investigation of ageing gray horse melanoma. J Anim Breed Genet 2000;117: 73–82.
25. Tuthil RJ, Clark RH, Levene A. Equine melanotic disease: a unique animal model for human dermal melanocytic disease. Lab Invest 1982;46:85A.
26. Sundström E, Komisarczuk AZ, Jiang L, et al. Identification of a melanocyte-specific, microphthalmia-associated transcription factor-dependent regulatory element in the intronic duplication causing hair graying and melanoma in horses. Pigment Cell Melanoma Res 2012;25:28–36.
27. Sundström E, Imsland F, Mikko S, et al. Copy number expansion of the STX17 duplication in melanoma tissue from Gray horses. BMC Genomics 2012;2(13): 365–77.
28. Campagne C, Julé S, Bernex F, et al. RACK1, a clue to the diagnosis of cutaneous melanomas in horses. BMC Vet Res 2012;8:95–103.
29. Sturm RA, Duffy DL, Box NF, et al. The role of melanocortin-1 receptor polymorphism in skin cancer risk phenotypes. Pigment Cell Res 2003;16:266–72.
30. Rieder S, Taourit S, Mariat D, et al. Mutations in the agouti (ASIP), the extension (MC1R), and the brown (TYRP1) loci and their association to coat color phenotypes in horses (*Equus caballus*). Mamm Genome 2001;12:450–5.
31. Smith AG, Luk N, Newton RA, et al. Melanocortin-1 receptor signaling markedly induces the expression of the NR4A nuclear receptor subgroup in melanocytic cells. J Biol Chem 2008;283:12564–70.
32. MacGillivray KC, Sweeney RW, Del Piero F. Metastatic melanoma in horses. J Vet Intern Med 2002;16:452–6.
33. Pulley LT, Stannard AA. Melanocytic tumor. In: Moulton JE, editor. Tumors in domestic animals. 3rd edition. Los Angeles (CA): University of California Press; 1990. p. 75–87.
34. Schott HC, Major MD, Grant BD, et al. Melanoma as a cause of spinal cord compression in two horses. J Am Vet Med Assoc 1990;196:1820–2.
35. Kirker-Head CA, Loeffler D, Held JP. Pelvic limb lameness due to malignant melanoma in a horse. J Am Vet Med Assoc 1985;186:1215–7.
36. Schöniger S, Summers BA. Equine skin tumours in 20 horses resembling three variants of human melanocytic naevi. Vet Dermatol 2009;20:165–73.
37. Traver DS, Moore JN, Thornburg LP, et al. Epidural melanoma causing posterior paresis in a horse. J Am Vet Med Assoc 1977;170:1400–3.
38. Milne JC. Malignant melanomas causing Horner's syndrome in a horse. Equine Vet J 1986;18:74–5.
39. Murray MJ, Cavey DM, Feldman BF, et al. Signs of sympathetic denervation associated with a thoracic melanoma in a horse. J Vet Intern Med 1997;11: 199–203.
40. Seltenhammer MH, Heere-Ress E, Brandt S, et al. Comparative histopathology of gray-horse-melanoma and human malignant melanoma. Pigment Cell Res 2004;17:674–81.
41. Rowe EL, Sullins KE. Excision as treatment of dermal melanomatosis in horses: 11 cases (1994-2000). J Am Vet Med Assoc 2004;225:94–6.
42. Stannard AA. The skin. In: Catcott EJ, editor. Equine medicine and surgery. 2nd edition. Wheaton (IL): American Veterinary Publications; 1972. p. 395–6.
43. Théon A. Radiation therapy in the horse. Vet Clin North Am Equine Pract 1998; 14(3):673–88.

44. Théon AP, Wilson WD, Magdesian KG, et al. Long-term outcome associated with intratumoral chemotherapy with cisplatin for cutaneous tumors in equidae: 573 cases (1995-2004). J Am Vet Med Assoc 2007;230:1506–13.

45. Hewes CA, Sullins KE. Use of cisplatin-containing biodegradable beads for treatment of cutaneous neoplasia in equidae: 59 cases (2000-2004). J Am Vet Med Assoc 2006;229:1617–22.

46. Stauffer PR. Evolving technology for thermal therapy of cancer. Int J Hyperthermia 2005;21:731–44.

47. Hoffman K, Krainer R, Shideler R. Radio-frequency current-induced hyperthermia for the treatment of equine sarcoid. Equine Pract 1983;5(7):24–31.

48. Smrkovski O, Koo Y, Kazemi R, et al. Performance characteristics of a conformal ultra-wideband multilayer applicator (CUMLA) for hyperthermia in veterinary patients. Vet Comp Oncol 2013;11:14–29.

49. Cemazar M, Tamzali Y, Sersa G, et al. Electrochemotherapy in veterinary oncology. J Vet Intern Med 2008;22:826–31.

50. Tamzali Y, Teissie J, Golzio M, et al. In: Jarm T, editor. Electrochemotherapy of equid cutaneous tumors: a 57 case retrospective study 1999–2005 [abstract 155]. New York: IFBME Proceedings; 2007. p. 610–3.

51. Spugnini EP, D' Alterio GL, Dotsinsky I, et al. Electrochemotherapy for the treatment of multiple melanomas in a horse. J Equine Vet Sci 2011;31:430–3.

52. Scacco L, Bolaffio C, Romano A, et al. Adjuvant electrochemotherapy increases local control in a recurring equine anal melanoma. J Eq Vet Sci 2013;33(8): 637–9.

53. Heinzerling LM, Feige K, Rieder S, et al. Tumor regression induced by intratumoral injection of DNA coding for human interleukin 12 into melanoma metastases in gray horses. J Mol Med (Berl) 2001;78:692–702.

54. Müller J, Feige K, Wunderlin P, et al. Double-blind placebo-controlled study with interleukin-18 and interleukin-12-encoding plasmid DNA shows antitumor effect in metastatic melanoma in gray horses. J Immunother 2011;34:58–64.

55. Trinchieri G. Interleukin-12: a proinflammatory cytokine with immunoregulatory functions that bridge innate resistance and antigen-specific adaptive immunity. Annu Rev Immunol 1995;13:251–76.

56. Rakhmilevich AL, Timmins JG, Janssen K, et al. Gene gun-mediated IL-12 gene therapy induces antitumor effects in the absence of toxicity: a direct comparison with systemic IL-12 protein therapy. J Immunother 1999;22:135–44.

57. Helfand SC, Soergel SA, MacWilliams PS, et al. Clinical and immunological effects of human recombinant interleukin-2 given by repetitive weekly infusion to normal dogs. Cancer Immunol Immunother 1994;39:84–92.

58. Ogden BE, Hill HR. Histamine regulates lymphocyte mitogenic responses through activation of specific H1 and H2 histamine receptors. Immunology 1980;41:107–14.

59. Brown AE, Badger AM, Poste G. The effect of cimetidine on immune cell functions and host response to tumors. In: Serrou B, Rosenfeld C, editors. Current concepts in human immunology and cancer immunomodulation. Amsterdam: Elsevier; 1982. p. 513.

60. Goetz TE, Ogilvie GK, Keegan KG, et al. Cimetidine for treatment of melanomas in three horses. J Am Vet Med Assoc 1990;196:449–52.

61. Bowers JR, Huntington PJ, Slocombe RF. Efficacy of cimetidine for therapy of skin tumors in horses—10 cases. Aust Vet J 1994;12:30.

62. Laus F, Cerquetella M, Paggi E, et al. Evaluation of cimetidine as a therapy for dermal melanomatosis in gray horses. Isr J Vet Med 2010;65:48–52.

63. Warnick LD, Graham ME, Valentine BA. Evaluation of cimetidine treatment for melanomas in seven horses. Equine Pract 1995;17:16–22.
64. Bergman PJ. Cancer immunotherapy. Vet Clin North Am Small Anim Pract 2010; 40:507–18.
65. Jeglum KA. Melanomas. In: Robinson NE, editor. Current therapy in equine medicine. 4th edition. Philadelphia: WB Saunders; 1997. p. 399–400.
66. Lembcke LM, Kania SA, Blackford JT, et al. Development of immunologic assays to measure response in horses vaccinated with xenogenic plasmid DNA encoding human tyrosinase. J Equine Vet Sci 2012;32:607–15.
67. Wang N, Hebert D. Tyrosinase maturation through the mammalian secretory pathway: bringing color to life. Pigment Cell Res 2006;19:3–18.
68. Phillips JC, Lembcke LM, Noltenius C, et al. Evaluation of tyrosinase expression in canine and equine melanocytic tumors. Am J Vet Res 2012;73:272–8.
69. USDA licenses DNA vaccine for treatment of melanoma in dogs. J Am Vet Med Assoc 2010;236:495.
70. Grosenbaugh DA, Leard AT, Bergman PJ, et al. Safety and efficacy of a xenogeneic DNA vaccine encoding for human tyrosinase as adjunctive treatment for oral malignant melanoma in dogs following surgical excision of the primary tumor. Am J Vet Res 2011;72:1631–8.
71. Phillips JC, Blackford JT, Lembcke LM, et al. Evaluation of needle free injection devices for intramuscular vaccination in horses. J Equine Vet Sci 2011;31: 738–43.

Heritable Equine Regional Dermal Asthenia

Ann Rashmir-Raven, DVM, MS

KEYWORDS

- Quarter Horse • Hereditary • Skin tearing • Collagen • HERDA • DNA testing

KEY POINTS

- Hereditary equine regional dermal asthenia (HERDA) is a form of Ehlers-Danlos syndrome that is most commonly seen in Quarter Horses, Appaloosas and American Paints.
- HERDA has an autosomal recessive mode of inheritance; DNA testing can establish normal, carrier and affected status.
- Affected horses are typically born normal and develop lesions within the first 2 years of life.
- More severely affected horses experience spontaneous skin sloughing and extensive lacerations, hematomas, and seromas from minor trauma, frequently resulting in disfiguring scars.
- Affected horses have a higher than expected incidence of corneal ulcers.
- Palliative therapy is available, but no curative treatment exists.

INTRODUCTION

Hereditary equine regional dermal asthenia (HERDA) is an autosomal recessive disorder of collagen observed primarily in Quarter Horses. It is a form of Ehlers-Danlos syndrome (EDS), which occurs in man and a variety of other species, such as cattle, sheep, dogs, cats, and mink. Ehlers-Danlos syndrome is a group of genetically heterogeneous connective tissue disorders that result from mutations in genes encoding various collagen types, enzymes that modify collagens, and other extracellular matrix proteins. When EDS occurs in animals, it is known by a variety of names, including *dermatosparaxis*, *cutaneous asthenia*, and *hyperelastosis cutis*.

HERDA has been extensively reported in the veterinary literature, beginning in 1978.[1–20] Because of the common practice of line breeding carrier horses, HERDA has recently become one of the most commonly reported inherited diseases in the

The author has nothing to disclose.
Department of Large Animal Clinical Sciences, Veterinary Medical Center, College of Veterinary Medicine, Michigan State University, 736 Wilson Road, Room A116, East Lansing, MI 48824, USA
E-mail address: rashmir@cvm.msu.edu

equine industry, and has been reported in Quarter Horses, Appaloosas, and American Paints in several countries, including the United States, Canada, Mexico, Brazil, England, France, and the Netherlands.

AUTOSOMAL MODE OF INHERITANCE

Heterozygous (N/Hrd) horses are carriers of the recessive Hrd allele, yet appear normal, without cutaneous signs of the disease. Horses that are homozygous for the recessive allele (Hrd/Hrd) are physically affected, and exhibit hyperextensible skin, cutaneous lesions, skin sloughing, and characteristic scarring. **Fig. 1** shows the typical pattern of inheritance for HERDA. When a carrier mare (N/Hrd) is bred to a carrier stallion (N/Hrd) there is a 25% chance that the foal will have HERDA (Hrd/Hrd), a 50% chance that the foal will be a carrier (N/Hrd) and a 25% chance that the foal will be totally normal (N/N). When a normal mare or stallion is bred to a carrier stallion or mare, a 50% chance exists that the foal will be a carrier, but a 0% chance that the foal will be affected. When an affected mare or stallion (Hrd/Hrd) is bred to a normal mare or stallion (N/N), all the foals will be carriers (N/Hrd). An affected foal can never be produced from a normal parent. Both parents must carry at least one copy of the HERDA gene.

SIGNIFICANCE WITHIN THE QUARTER HORSE INDUSTRY

Although cutting horses are most commonly affected, pleasure, reining, working cow, and foundation bred horses are also affected. In cutting horses alone, 3 of the 10 leading lifetime sires (leading lifetime cutting horse sires, all ages, all divisions[6]) are confirmed carriers. As of 2012, these 3 sires alone have produced 5792 total registered offspring, including performing and nonperforming offspring. By virtue of HERDA's autosomal recessive mode of inheritance, one-half of these offspring (2896) are HERDA carriers or affected animals. The total lifetime earnings of these 3 carriers is $109,008,304; an average earning of $31,583 per performance offspring.

Carrier to carrier mating:

	N	Hrd
N	N/N	N/Hrd
Hrd	N/Hrd	Hrd/Hrd

N = Normal allele   Hrd = Abnormal allele

Normal horse mated to carrier:

	N	N
N	N/N	N/N
Hrd	N/Hrd	N/Hrd

N = Normal allele   Hrd = Abnormal allele

Fig. 1. Typical pattern of inheritance for HERDA showing matings of carrier to carrier and carrier to normal horse.

In comparison, the 7 remaining noncarrier stallions in the top 10 lifetime sires made $152,148,156 in offspring earnings, accounting for an average earning of $27,249 per performance offspring, which is significantly lower (−$4334.00) than that for carriers. In addition, the top 3 carrier sire's earnings represent 42% of the total income generated by the top 10 horses. Previous work has shown that the income generated by the top carrier stallions has been increasing approximately 5% faster than for noncarrier stallions since 1998 (**Fig. 2**). The prevalence of the HERDA mutation in elite performance horses has raised the question whether the HERDA mutation or a closely linked gene confers a performance advantage. Alternatively, these horses may simply be outstanding performers irrespective of the mutation.

CLINICAL SIGNS

The hallmark of the disease is the presence of multiple areas of loose, stretchy, hyperextensible skin that is not well attached to the horse. Lesional areas may range from the size of a dime to the involvement of almost the entire surface area of the horse (**Figs. 3** and **4**). Fragile skin, spontaneous skin sloughing (**Fig. 5**), and disfiguring scars are common (**Fig. 6**). Although subtle signs of the condition, such as a loose mane or an unusual amount of joint flexibility, may be present at birth, most commonly HERDA is not noticed until skin lesions develop at approximately 18 to 24 months of age. Some affected individuals do not develop lesions until 4 or 5 years of age. The occasional horse is so mildly affected that it seems to never develop typical lesions and, despite the presence of loose stretchy skin, presents a diagnostic challenge. Usually, when the horse enters training, lesions become pronounced because the saddle sits over the most severely affected skin. Large tissue sloughs and hematomas (**Fig. 7**) may occur at this time. Some horses become painful and display significant changes in behavior and attitude. Commonly, by the time the disease is finally diagnosed, considerable financial and emotional investments have been made.

Aside from minimizing trauma, no treatment is known. The heritable nature of the disease makes these horses unsuitable for breeding. As a result, a large number of elite-bred animals are humanely destroyed each year.

The severity, age of onset, and extent of skin lesions in HERDA vary considerably from horse to horse. **Fig. 8** shows a 6-year-old mare that, despite having classic signs of HERDA and a positive DNA test (Hrd/Hrd), successfully competes in reining. She has

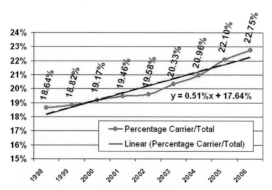

Fig. 2. Percentage of carrier (N/Hr) sire lifetime earnings relative to total 100 sire lifetime earnings (1998 through 2006). Carrier's earnings increase approximately 0.5% per year compared with normal horses ($P<.0001$).

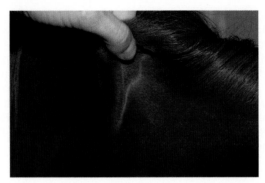

Fig. 3. An example of loose, stretchy skin on a 6-year-old Quarter Horse stallion with HERDA.

one small lesion just cranial to her loin and an excessively loose mane. **Fig. 9** shows a 6-year-old pasture-bred breeding stallion with much more severe skin lesions.

In addition to heritable factors, environmental influences are believed to be significant. The most common HERDA horse lesions occur over the dorsal midline, where both heat and ultraviolet (UV) light are more intense. Lesions generally improve when the horse is restricted to a stall environment for 2 to 4 weeks. HERDA horses that are continually maintained indoors and out of the sun have fewer problems than those maintained outside. The authors' observations also indicate that UV fly sheets, winter months, and northern climates are associated with a decrease in the severity of the condition. Both temperature and UV light are believed to play a role in disease progression. In humans, elevations in temperature and UV light are known to disrupt the dermal extracellular matrix by inducing matrix metalloproteinases (ie, collagenase). Because HERDA horse collagen is more soluble, loosely bound, and disorganized than that of normal horses, it may be more susceptible to the effects of enzymatic degradation. Anecdotal evidence suggests that HERDA lesions are also influenced by hormonal status. The most severely affected horses encountered thus far are intact male horses. However, stallions may be more likely to traumatize their skin. The severity of skin lesions has also been noted to wax and wane with pregnancy in some animals.

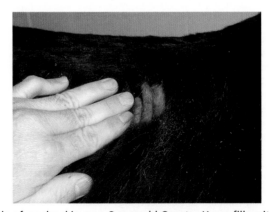

Fig. 4. An example of mushy skin on a 2-year-old Quarter Horse filly with HERDA.

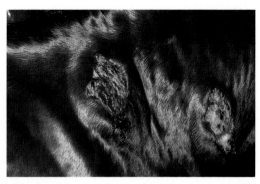

Fig. 5. Spontaneous skin sloughing in a 6-year-old Quarter Horse stallion, typical of a horse severely affected with HERDA.

DERMAL FINDINGS

A study of the skin from 10 HERDA horses and 6 control horses showed that compared with normal horses, HERDA horses exhibited a 2- to 3-fold reduction in tensile strength and modulus of elasticity. These findings were consistent over several body regions. In addition, in a study of 13 HERDA horses and 12 control horses, HERDA horses exhibited significantly higher amounts of total soluble collagen in their skin than unaffected horses. Another published report of the biochemical properties of collagen from patients with HERDA detected increased acid soluble collagen. Types I and III collagens demonstrated their expected molecular weights. However, detailed comparison using high-resolution SDS-PAGE acrylamide gel electrophoresis, peptide mapping, and other techniques that have been useful in characterizing collagen disorders of humans have not been reported in horses.

OCULAR FINDINGS

One study of 28 HERDA horses and 291 non-HERDA horses evaluated over a 4-year period showed an increased incidence of corneal ulceration and a decreased corneal thickness in HERDA horses compared with non-HERDA control horses. Abnormal collagen fibril arrangement was also present in the corneas of HERDA horses, but not in the corneas of controls.

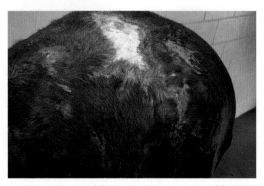

Fig. 6. Disfiguring scars on a 5-year-old Quarter Horse mare with HERDA.

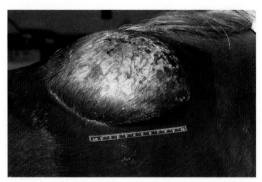

Fig. 7. Large hematoma on a 3-year-old Quarter Horse gelding with HERDA.

MUSCULOSKELETAL

Similar to humans with EDS who often experience joint pain and osteoarthritis, increasing evidence suggests that HERDA horses are at increased risk for osteoarthritis. A pilot study of articular cartilage from the joints of 5 consecutive juvenile horses with HERDA showed gross and histologic evidence of osteoarthritic lesions. Furthermore, chondrocyte cultures from these same horses had increased matrix metalloproteinase activity and spontaneously produced greater prostaglandin E2 (PGE2) than chondrocytes from normal horses (41,000-fold). Because the increased PGE2 activity was responsive to treatment with both phenylbutazone and a glucosamine and chondroitin product, Cosequin, Cosequin is often recommended for the prevention and treatment of osteoarthritis in HERDA horses and has anecdotally led to some improvements in skin.

Tendonoligamentous structures have been shown to be weaker in horses with HERDA. In a study that evaluated the suspensory ligament and superficial and deep digital flexor tendons from the forelimbs of 6 HERDA horses and 6 age-matched controls, the HERDA horses' tendinoligamentous structures had a significantly lower tensile strength than normal. The joints in HERDA horses can be profoundly hypermobile compared with age-matched control Quarter Horses (**Figs. 10** and **11**). The altered

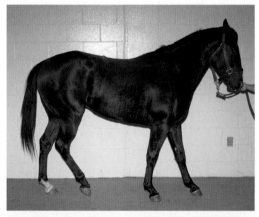

Fig. 8. Mildly affected 6-year-old mare that actively competes in reining. She has one small lesion just cranial to her loin.

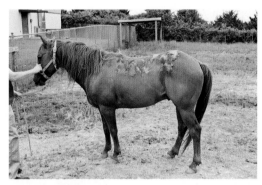

Fig. 9. Severely affected 6-year-old stallion.

biomechanics in HERDA tendons and ligaments, coupled with joint hypermobility, has added to the speculation that the HERDA mutation in heterozygous (carrier) horses enhances flexibility and provides a competitive advantage in the athletic disciplines to which the mutation has segregated.

IMMUNE FUNCTION

Anecdotal evidence of increased susceptibility to bacterial or parasitic infections has been reported in HERDA horses. Cyclophilin B contributes to the regulation of integrin-mediated adhesion of T lymphocytes into an inflammatory site. Therefore, HERDA horses may be more susceptible to certain types of infections or cancer. Two cases

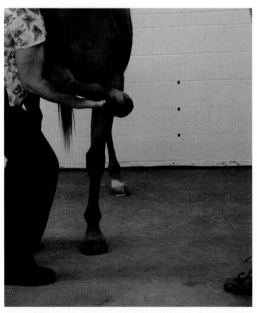

Fig. 10. Hypermobility in an 8-year-old horse with HERDA. This horse had been ridden for 6 years before being tested for HERDA. Other than the presence of loose, stretchy skin, the horse had no other dermal lesions.

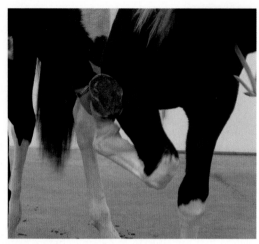

Fig. 11. Hypermobility in a yearling Paint with HERDA.

of disseminated squamous cell carcinoma (SCC) have been reported in HERDA horses. Failure of immune surveillance due to T-cell malfunction as a result of the HERDA cyclophilin B mutation, along with exposure to UV light, chronic inflammation, and poorly formed dermal collagen, were believed to be responsible for the development of SCC at the wound sites, and subsequent pulmonary metastasis. Alternatively, the increased metastatic potential of the SCC in the 2 reported cases may have been from increased vulnerability to matrix metalloproteinase digestion caused by the increased solubility of collagen, resulting in an increase in angiogenesis and tumor invasiveness. Neither wound-site SCC nor pulmonary metastasis is a common occurrence in normal horses, although SCC has, rarely, been reported in association with chronic ulcers or burn scars.

DEFECTIVE COLLAGEN CROSS-LINKING

Because HERDA shares several clinical similarities to Ehlers-Danlos type VIA, in which the urinary concentrations of the collagen pyridinium cross-links deoxypyridinoline (DPD) and pyridinoline (PYD) are used to diagnose the disease, the ratios of DPD:PYD in the urine, skin, and other tissues were evaluated in 19 HERDA horses and 39 controls. Horses with HERDA had significantly higher DPD and DPD:PYD ratios in the urine, skin, and other tissues compared with control horses. The concentrations of PYD and hydroxylysine in the skin of horses with HERDA were significantly lower than in control horses. Lysine and total pyridinium cross-links were not significantly different between groups. Supplementing HERDA horses with lysine was originally proposed as a potential treatment for this disease, with some HERDA horse owners feeling strongly about its benefits.

HISTOLOGY

Although the histologic changes associated with HERDA are considered controversial by some clinicians, histology can lead to a presumptive diagnosis, which can be confirmed with DNA testing. A diagnostic biopsy is technically more difficult to perform on HERDA skin, but is critical to providing an informative sample. Because the skin of HERDA horses naturally splits between the superficial and deep dermis, complete biopsy samples containing the deep dermis are difficult to obtain, and the submission of just the upper layer of the lesion for histology will render the biopsy useless. In addition, HERDA skin samples are friable and can separate during processing. Clear histologic differences between nonlesional skin in horses with HERDA and normal skin from unaffected horses may not be apparent. Several lesions of HERDA that seem to be unique may not be apparent in all superficial biopsies of skin. Early lesions of HERDA show mild thinning of collagen bundles (hyperextensible areas) in the mid dermis. As the lesions progress, increased space between collagen bundles, loss of bundle compactness, and collagen bundle fraying are observed. In more advanced lesions (depending on the stage of resolution), dense inflammation or collagenous connective tissue seems to expand easily, filling defects in the intermediate layer of the dermis.

In areas of chronically detached skin, collagen bundles become frayed with the wear between the superficial and deep layers. In the absence of infection or perforation of the skin, HERDA lesions have a paucity of inflammatory infiltrate and show little evidence of physiologic repair. Biopsies taken from areas in which the skin has been perforated often show extensive inflammation and fibrovascular proliferation that can obscure the more characteristic diagnostic changes.

Histologic findings from the junction of lesional and nonlesional skin, showing fraying or separation of the intermediate dermis, support a presumptive diagnosis that is otherwise made on compatible clinical presentation and pedigree. Care and experience are required to differentiate artifactual from pathologic separation of the dermis in punch biopsies. A study by White and colleagues[19] showed that pathologists differ in their ability to identify characteristic changes, confirming the need to have biopsy samples interpreted by pathologists with proven expertise in this area. It also suggests that DNA testing is a superior method of diagnosis. Any suspicious findings on histopathology should be confirmed with DNA testing.

MUTATION ORIGINS

The gene can be traced back to its origin with the Quarter Horse sire Poco Bueno. Of the 5000 horses that were DNA tested at Cornell University (including 155 affected horses), all heterozygous carriers trace back to this prominent sire, and all homozygous-affected horses exhibit parental consanguinity to Poco Bueno. In a study in which 75 pedigrees of affected horses were evaluated, 100% exhibited consanguinity to Poco Bueno within 7 generations. Evidence of the mutation being passed on by King P234, Poco Bueno's sire, through offspring other than Poco Bueno has not yet emerged through testing. Evidence of the mutation having originated with Miss Taylor, Poco Buenos' dam, remains controversial.

Poco Bueno's genetic contribution has been multiplied through many generations, so the opportunity for carrier-to-carrier mating has increased. Poco Bueno sired 405 American Quarter Horse Association (AQHA)–registered, first-generation foals, 50% of which would be carriers. His second generation included 537 foals, 25% of which would be carriers, and his third generation included 1352 foals, 12.5% of which would be carriers. These first 3 generations from Poco Bueno alone account for approximately 500 horses that had a probability of carrying the HERDA gene. Of the 3.2 million registered Quarter Horses that are still alive, more than 1.7 million trace back to Poco Bueno. This lineage is also considered the fastest growing segment of the Quarter Horse population.

Within the general Quarter Horse population, the disease is much more prevalent in the cutting horse industry. However, carriers have also been identified in other performance disciplines. The reining, working cow, and pleasure horse industries all have top-ranked performance horses that are confirmed carriers. The offspring of these horses often excel in more than one discipline, and as more carriers are produced, more disciplines will be impacted.

Selection pressure for performance traits associated with Poco Bueno may have resulted in higher inbreeding coefficients in the general performance population, in addition to contributing to the increasing number of affected horses presently observed. Linebreeding and inbreeding programs are commonly used in performance horse bloodlines and are used to maintain a degree of genetic relationship to an outstanding ancestor. Although animals with performance advantages can be produced, the increased inbreeding results in a higher frequency of hereditary abnormalities from an increase in homozygosity of recessive genes. Within the general Quarter Horse population, the HERDA carrier frequency is 3.5%. However, cutting horses have a significantly higher carrier frequency of 28%, indicating that the disease is much more prevalent within the cutting horse industry. Western pleasure horses and working-cow horses have published carrier frequency rates of 12.8% and 11.5% respectively. For reining horses, the carrier frequency is likely not far behind. The overall carrier frequency in American Paint horses is 1.7%, which is approximately one-half the frequency of the general Quarter Horse population. Because the disease is becoming increasingly more common, selective breeding based on DNA testing is recommended to reduce the number of animals that have HERDA and the financial and emotional losses incurred by HERDA horse owners.

The AQHA is requiring all stallions breeding 25 or more mares to be tested for HERDA as of 2014. In 2015, all stallions breeding 1 or more mares will be required to be tested as a part of the registration process. Test results will be recorded on horse registration and available to all AQHA members through an online database. Genetic testing is a simple, inexpensive procedure that requires approximately 40 mane or tail hairs be pulled so that the root is visible on the hair shaft. Information is available at http://www.vgl.ucdavis.edu/.

GENETIC MUTATION DESCRIBED

A homozygosity mapping approach identified a nonsynonymous single nucleotide polymorphism (SNP) in the cyclophilin B gene with the HERDA phenotype, indicating that the disease is caused by a mutation in the cyclophilin B (PPIB) gene. Functional studies have confirmed this. CYPB is a member of the peptidyl-prolyl *cis*-trans isomerase family of proteins, which catalyze prolyl-containing bonds in procollagen to the trans configuration. This trans configuration is required to form the triple-helical collagen molecule. Conventionally viewed as the primary rate-limiting enzyme in fibrillar collagen synthesis, CYPB also has critical functions in procollagen trafficking, processing, and chain association. The HERDA mutation does not alter prolyl isomerization activity of CYPB, but delays collagen folding and secretion and modifies a region of CYPB that identifies improperly folded proteins in the endoplasmic reticulum. These events are presumed to alter collagen organization.

DIFFERENTIAL DIAGNOSES

Trauma to a normal horse can easily cause wounds similar to those seen with HERDA; however, stretchy, loose skin and other signs such as joint hypermobility are not generally present. Junctional epidermolysis bullosa (JEB) can be confused with HERDA but has not been reported in Quarter Horses and, unlike HERDA, occurs at birth. JEB affects Belgian foals and is occasionally seen in Warmbloods. Affected foals develop erosions and ulceration of the skin and mucous membranes in the first few days of life. Dental abnormalities are another characteristic of the disease, including irregularly serrated edges and enamel pits on incisors and cheek teeth, and the premature eruption of the teeth, with the central incisors and premolars present at birth. The disease is invariably fatal as a result of secondary sepsis, and euthanasia is essential in confirmed cases.

A blistering skin disorder that can be confused with HERDA and is similar to JEB has been observed in foals of other breeds, including American Saddlebreds and Appaloosas. In American Saddlebreds, the disease is known as *epitheliogenesis imperfecta* and is caused by an unknown but distinct genetic defect. Other skin fragility syndromes in foals include various forms of vasculitis and sepsis, with or without platelet anomalies, which are often treatable. Again, these diseases most commonly occur in animals much younger than those with HERDA.

Pemphigus foliaceus, lupus, drug eruptions, and other immune-mediated diseases can occasionally be confused with HERDA. Some of these occur in same-age horses and may show similar signs, although the course of the diseases is different, as is the lack of the stretchy, mushy skin.

In the author's experience, the disease that is most frequently mistaken for HERDA is severe dermatophilosis in weanling, yearling, or 2-year-old Quarter Horses. Dermatophilosis is caused by the gram-positive actinomycete *Dermatophilus congolensis*, which is a common source of bacterial dermatitis in the horse. The dorsally distributed hair loss and skin sloughing that is common with dermatophilosis is incorrectly assumed to be HERDA by some horse owners (**Fig. 12**). It is important to note that HERDA-like disease occurs in a variety of horse breeds (including Quarter Horses) without the PPIB mutation. In the absence of the PPIB mutation the disease is simply referred to as Ehlers-Danlos syndrome.

MANAGEMENT/PROGNOSIS

Management of HERDA-affected individuals includes minimizing trauma, careful wound management, and restriction from heat and sunlight. Nutritional status is addressed to ensure an optimal diet. Special attention is given to dietary copper and vitamin C content, because they are cofactors in the metabolism of collagen.

Mildly affected horses may be ridden, with a percentage of these horses being competition-sound. With excellent care, some individuals can live a good number of years; several have lived into their late 20s. Because of the availability of DNA testing

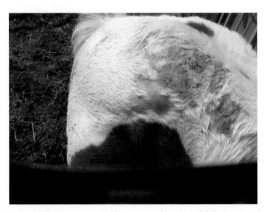

Fig. 12. A weanling colt with *Dermatophilus congolensis,* which is occasionally mistaken for HERDA.

and the greater awareness of the disease, HERDA is being diagnosed earlier in horses. As a result, most horses with HERDA are humanely destroyed by 3 years of age because they are unsound for both riding and breeding, although unfortunately, this assumption can be the source of some confusion. Veterinarians and horse owners alike occasionally assume that when they see an older horse with stretchy skin and/ or a horse that has been successfully ridden, it cannot have HERDA. Mildly affected horses can be ridden and shown, which calls into question the fate of young foals that are DNA tested before the onset of clinical symptoms.

Owners who are interested in maintaining horses with HERDA should consider the following recommendations:

- Minimize exposure to intense sunlight and heat as much as practical. Nighttime turnout is recommended, as is UV fly sheet protection.
- Minimize wounds whenever possible through appropriate fencing and stabling; turnout with well-matched, gentle horses or restrict HERDA horses to individual turnout. Treat all wounds gently and avoid significant pressure when cleaning or hosing.
- Avoid caustic agents.
- Establish drainage in hematomas early, otherwise these can become large.
- Attempt to suture deeper, penetrating wounds; suturing common, superficial wounds of horses with HERDA is rarely successful.
- Handle the horse often to ensure ease of wound treatment when necessary.
- Ensure excellent fly control to minimize self-trauma.
- Use a fan in the stall to minimize heat and insect exposure.
- Understand that cooler weather seems to be beneficial for horses with HERDA, as is the longer hair coat that accompanies winter months.

NUTRITION

Adequate protein is an important component in nutrition. Appropriate attention to trace minerals is needed; copper, selenium, and vitamin C are of particular importance. Cosequin or a similar chondroitin sulfate and glucosamine product may prove useful in select cases.

SUMMARY

The high prevalence and tremendous economic value of Quarter Horses that carry the genetic defect responsible for HERDA assure that this disease will be around for many more generations. As has been shown repeatedly with other heritable equine diseases, even with the advent of DNA testing to identify HERDA carriers, the popularity of these lineages guarantees that horses both heterozygous and homozygous for the trait will continue to be produced. The recognition of more subtly affected animals will be an important aspect of equine practice in the future. Managed breeding strategy of horses or embryos, based on DNA testing, is the only method currently available to minimize the production of affected horses.

No treatment exists, although minimizing exposure to sunlight and trauma, coupled with appropriate dietary supplementation and gentle wound care, may improve the quality of life of affected horses and give some affected animals significant longevity. Mildly affected horses may still be ridden, with a percentage of these being competition-sound. The incidence of affected but competition-sound individuals is not currently known, but this again brings into question the concerns over the fate of individuals that test homozygous for the disease at a young age.

ACKNOWLEDGMENTS

The author gratefully acknowledges the support of Drs Melinda Poole, Nena Winand, Sharon Black, Sabrina Brounts, Richard Hopper, Peter Ryan, Cate Mochal, Jesse Grady, Robin Fontenot, Jim Cooley, Steve Elder, Narelle Stubbs, Hilary Clayton and Carmelita Frondoza; Ms Sally Tipton; and Mr Ronnie Braswell. The author wishes to acknowledge the tremendous support provided by Iron Rose Ranch, Ms. Marcia Lane and the American Quarter Horse Association. In addition, the material presented in this article would not be available without the help of many other veterinarians and horse owners who have provided horses, samples, and information over the past 16 years.

REFERENCES

1. Bachinger HP. The influence of peptidyl-prolyl cis-trans isomerase on the in vitro folding of type III collagen. J Biol Chem 1987;262:17144–8.
2. Bowser JE, Elder S, Rashmir-Raven AM, et al. Tensile properties in collagen rich tissues of Quarter Horses with hereditary equine regional dermal asthenia (HERDA). Equine Vet J 2013. http://dx.doi.org/10.1111/evj.12110.
3. Bridges CH, McMullan WC. Dermatosparaxis in quarter horses. In: Proceedings of the 35th Annual Meeting of the American College of Veterinary Pathologists. Toronto: American College of Veterinary Pathologists; 1984. p. 12.
4. Brounts SH, Rashmir-Raven AM, Black SS. Zonal dermal separation: a distinctive histopathological lesion associated with hyperelastosis cutis in a Quarter Horse. Vet Dermatol 2001;12:219–24.
5. Dorris ML, Rashmir-Raven AM, Heinecke LF, et al. Increased metalloproteinase activity in chondrocytes from articular cartilage of horses with Hereditary Equine Regional Dermal Asthenia. J Vet Intern Med 2011;25:632–767.
6. Available at: http://equistat.com/.
7. Gardner LC, Rashmir-Raven AM, Heinecke LF, et al. Articular cartilage from horses afflicted with Hereditary Equine Regional Dermal Asthenia (HERDA) exhibits osteoarthritic lesions and isolated chondrocytes produce high levels of the pro-inflammatory mediator prostaglandin E2. J Vet Intern Med 2011;25:632–767.
8. Grady JG, Elder SH, Ryan PL, et al. Biomechanical and molecular characteristics of hereditary equine regional dermal asthenia in Quarter Horses. Vet Dermatol 2009;20:591–9.
9. Hardy MH, Fisher KR, Vrablic OE, et al. An inherited connective tissue disease in the horse. Lab Invest 1988;59:253–6.
10. Ishikawa Y, Vranka JA, Boudko SP, et al. The mutation in cyclophilin B that causes hyperelastosis cutis in the American Quarter Horse does not affect peptidyl-prolyl cis-trans isomerase activity, but shows altered cyclophilin B-protein interactions and affects collagen folding. J Biol Chem 2012;287: 22253–65.
11. Lerner DJ, McCracken MD. Hyperelastosis cutis in 2 horses. J Equine Med Surg 1978;2:350–2.
12. Mochal CA, Miller WW, Cooley AJ, et al. Ocular findings in Quarter Horses with hereditary equine regional dermal asthenia. J Am Vet Med Assoc 2010;237: 304–10.
13. Rashmir-Raven AM, Winand NJ, Read RW, et al. Equine hyperelastosis cutis update. In: Am Assoc Equine Pract 2004;50:47–50.
14. Stannard AA. Stannard's illustrated equine dermatology notes. Vet Dermatol 2000;11:211–5.

15. Swiderski CE, Pasquali M, Schwarz L, et al. The Ratio of Urine Deoxypyridinoline to Pyridinoline Identifies Horses with HyperElastosis Cutis (a.ka. Hereditary Equine Regional Dermal Aesthenia, HERDA). JVIM 2006;20:802.

16. Tipton SG, Anderson JD, Smith TS, et al. Epidemiologic and economic study of hyperelastosis cutis/HERDA in the Quarter Horse cutting industry [abstract]. J Anim Sci 2008;86(Suppl) [abstract 548].

17. Tryon RC, Penedo MC, McCue ME, et al. Evaluation of allele frequencies of inherited disease genes in subgroups of American Quarter Horses. J Am Vet Med Assoc 2009;234:120–5.

18. Tryon RC, White SD, Bannasch DL. Homozygosity mapping approach identifies a missense mutation in equine cyclophilin B (PPIB) associated with HERDA in American Quarter Horses. Genomics 2007;90:93–102.

19. White SD, Affolter VK, Bannasch DL, et al. Hereditary equine regional dermal asthenia ('hyperelastosis cutis') in 50 horses: clinical, histologic, immunohisto-logic and ultrastructural findings. Vet Dermatol 2004;15:207–17.

20. White SD, Affolter VK, Schulteiss PC. Clinical and pathological findings in a HERDA-affected foal for 1.5 years of life. Vet Dermatol 2007;18:36–40.

Donkey Dermatology

Stephen D. White, DVM

KEYWORDS

- Donkey • Dermatology • Skin • Dermatoses

KEY POINTS

- The most important bacterial skin infection on a worldwide basis is that caused by the actinomycete *Dermatophilus congolensis*.
- *Trichophyton verrucosum* and *Trichophyton mentagrophytes* have been reported as causing alopecia and scaling in donkeys.
- Molluscum contagiosum has been reported in donkeys.
- *Habronema* sp, lice, biting flies, and *Chorioptes* sp can all afflict donkeys, as they do horses. Anecdotally, cutaneous habronemiasis has been thought to cause more severe lesions (in general) in donkeys and mules than in horses.
- Sarcoids are the most common cutaneous tumor in donkeys.

Donkeys (*Equus asinus*) are a species used throughout the world primarily as beasts of burden, but occasionally for other functions, as a meat source or as pets. Although closely related to horses and zebras (they can produce sterile hybrids with both), they have some unique features of their own with regard to dermatologic disease. This article attempts to briefly highlight some of the various dermatoses seen or reported in donkeys, as well as some comparisons with horses when prevalence, presentation, or treatment may differ.

Vocabulary: in English, a male donkey is called a "jack," a female is a "jenny," and a castrated male a "cut-jack" or a "donkey gelding."

CONGENITAL DERMATOSES

As has been reported in horses, junctional epidermal bullosa has been noted in a donkey foal.[1] The disease was characterized by ulceration of large areas of the skin on the legs and ears. Interestingly, the foal was noted to be "normal" at birth. The progression of the disease is fatal.

Department of Medicine and Epidemiology, School of Veterinary Medicine, Veterinary Medical Teaching Hospital, University of California, 1 Shields Avenue, Davis, CA 95616, USA
E-mail address: sdwhite@ucdavis.edu

Vet Clin Equine 29 (2013) 703–708
http://dx.doi.org/10.1016/j.cveq.2013.08.002
0749-0739/13/$ – see front matter © 2013 Elsevier Inc. All rights reserved.

BACTERIAL DISEASE

Perhaps the most important bacterial skin infection on a worldwide basis is that caused by the actinomycete *Dermatophilus congolensis*. Antibiotics, such as trimethoprim-sulfamethoxazole, as well as topical washings, are the recommended treatment. Interestingly, dosing intervals for *intravenous* administration of trimethoprim-sulfamethoxazole in horses may not be appropriate for use in donkeys or mules. Donkeys eliminate the drugs rapidly compared with horses.[2] Thus, dosing intervals probably need to be more frequent in donkeys than in horses. The same has been found in preliminary research for amikacin, oxytetracycline, and the beta-lactam antibiotics. The opposite seems to be the case for the fluoroquinolone marbofloxacin. Another antibiotic in the same class, norfloxacin, should be avoided in donkeys, because of neurologic signs when injected intravenously, swelling at intramuscular injection sites, and poor bioavailability when given orally.[3]

Other bacterial skin infections, such as those caused by staphylococcal species or *Corynebacterium pseudotuberculosis* (**Fig. 1**), are also occasionally seen in donkeys.

FUNGAL INFECTIONS

Trichophyton verrucosum and *Trichophyton mentagrophytes* have been reported as causing alopecia and scaling in donkeys.[4]

Deeper fungal infections, such as those caused by *Sporothrix schenckii*, *Cryptococcosus* sp, *Histoplasma capsulatum* (North American histoplasmosis), and *H capsulatum var farciminosum* ("farcy": the cause of equine epizootic lymphangitis in east Africa) have been reported in donkeys.[5–9] The latter fungus especially has yielded a number of articles on both clinical signs and diagnoses. In general, deep fungal infections present clinically with nodules and ulcers, often with a purulent exudate. Thickened ("corded") lymphatics may be noted, especially in *H capsulatum var farciminosum* infections. Sporotrichosis seems to have a tendency to affect the inguinal area and medial aspect of the rear legs (**Fig. 2**A), although other areas of the body may also be affected (**Fig. 2**B). Diagnosis may be achieved by cytology, culture, or histopathology.

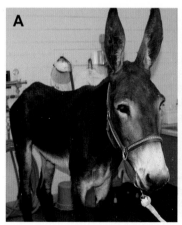 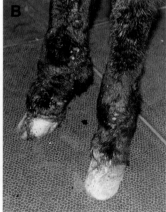

Fig. 1. (*A*) A 7-year-old jenny with weight loss due to internal abscesses caused by *Corynebacterium pseudotuberculosis*. (*B*) The same donkey as in (*A*). Purulent/hemorrhagic abscesses on both rear legs, caused by *C pseudotuberculosis*. Note edema of legs ("stocking up").

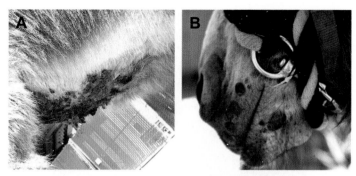

Fig. 2. (A) A 5-year-old jenny with inguinal ulceration and crusts, due to *Sporothrix schenckii* infection. (B) The same donkey as in (A). Ulcerative nodules on muzzle, due to *S schenckii* infection.

Treatment with oral potassium iodide (KI) and fluconazole may be helpful in controlling, if not curing, these infections.[8,9] Reported dosage regimens for KI are 0.5 to 2.0 mg/kg daily for 2.5 years[9] or 40 mg/kg daily for 10 days[8]; the dosage for fluconazole is 1 mg/kg daily for 2 years.[9]

VIRAL INFECTIONS

Molluscum contagiosum has been reported in donkeys.[10] Like horses, donkeys are susceptible to the mucosal viruses, such as vesicular stomatitis.

PARASITIC INFESTATIONS

Habronema sp, lice, biting flies, and *Chorioptes* sp can all afflict donkeys, as they do horses. Anecdotally, cutaneous habronemiasis has been thought to cause more severe lesions (in general) in donkeys and mules than in horses.

A form of cutaneous onchocerciasis is seen in donkeys in Africa and possibly in other nearby areas, which causes severe ulceration in the withers and neck region; it is the adult parasite (sometimes extractable by hand) that causes this problem. The possible causative species is *Onchocerca raillieti*. Interestingly, ivermectin has been reported as having both greater and lesser gastrointestinal absorption in donkeys than in horses. This awaits more clarifying studies.[3]

Donkeys are apparently more susceptible to infestation with the parasite *Besnoitia bennetti* than horses, judging from the reports in the literature.[11–15] This organism is the same species that afflicts cattle, and is closely related to *Besnoitia tarandi*, which afflicts reindeer (*Rangifer tarandus*).[11] The disease presents as nodules (cysts) on the skin, nares, and sclera. Scaling on the skin may be noted. Multiple donkeys in a herd may be affected.[14,15] Diagnosis may be by histopathology, serologic testing, and polymerase chain reaction.[14,15] Unfortunately there is no known effective treatment.

Donkeys, like horses, can be afflicted with a hypersensitivity to *Culicoides* spp.[16]

NEOPLASIA

Sarcoids are the most common cutaneous tumor in donkeys (**Fig. 3**). Donkeys (particularly male donkeys) have a higher incidence of sarcoids than is seen in horses. As in horses and zebras, a number of researchers have been able to isolate bovine papilloma virus DNA from sarcoids of donkeys.[17–19]

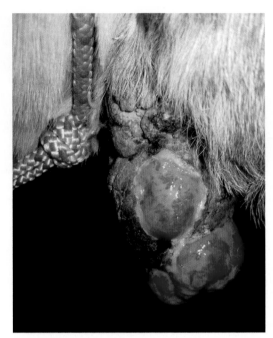

Fig. 3. A 5-year-old jack with ulcerated verrucous sarcoid.

MISCELLANEOUS DISEASES

Donkeys have been described with pemphigus foliaceous. In one jenny, the disease occurred during, then regressed after 2 of its 5 pregnancies.[20]

Donkeys have been reported with pituitary pars intermedia dysfunction, also known as equine Cushing disease.[21] The initial dosage of pergolide reported as effective in treatment is 0.002 mg/kg per day.[22]

Equine sarcoidosis has been seen in at least one donkey (Dr Wayne Rosenkrantz, personal communication, Anaheim, CA, December 2012).

"'Seedy toe' is by definition an abnormal separation at the white line into which foreign material frequently gets wedged and forced into the depth of the hoof wall. Infection is common. It can arise from laminitis or overgrowth or management problems and is usually regarded as a preventable disease entity" (Professor Derek Knottenbelt, personal communication via e-mail, January 2012). Based on research done at the Donkey Sanctuary (www.thedonkeysanctuary.org.uk), the donkey hoof wall is capable of much greater absorption of water than the hoof wall of the horse. This is presumably an advantage in retaining scarce water in the arid environment where donkeys evolved, but is a detriment in moist climates or wet stables, such that the hooves may be prone to white line disease (Dr Alex Thiemann, personal communication via e-mail, October 2011). This latter disease is defined as "a keratinolytic process that originates on the solar surface of the hoof."[23]

ACKNOWLEDGMENTS

The author is extremely grateful to the advice given him on skin disease in donkeys from the following colleagues: Drs Patrick Bourdeau, Derek Knottenbelt, Marianne M. Sloet van Oldruitenborgh-Oostrbaan, and Alex Thiemann.

REFERENCES

1. Sloet van Oldruitenborgh-Oostrbaan M, Boord M. Equine dermatology workshop. In: Thoday KL, Foil CS, Bond R, editors. Advances in veterinary dermatology, vol. 4. Oxford (United Kingdom): Blackwell Science; 2002. p. 286–90.
2. Peck KE, Matthews NS, Taylor TS, et al. Pharmacokinetics of sulfamethoxazole and trimethoprim in donkeys, mules, and horses. Am J Vet Res 2002;63: 349–53.
3. Grosenbaugh DA, Reinemeyerr CR, Figueiredo MD. Pharmacology and therapeutics in donkeys. Equine Vet Educ 2011;23:523–30.
4. Abdalla WG, Suliman EA, Gabbar AE. A report on *Trichophyton verrucosum* in donkeys in the Sudan. Sudan J Vet Res 2005;20:83–5.
5. Cooper VL, Kennedy GA, Kruckenberg SM, et al. Histoplasmosis in a miniature Sicilian burro. J Vet Diagn Invest 1994;6:499–501.
6. Irizarry-Rovira AR, Kaufman L, Christian JA, et al. Diagnosis of sporotrichosis in a donkey using direct fluorescein-labeled antibody testing. J Vet Diagn Invest 2000;12:180–3.
7. Khodakaram-Tafti A, Dehghani S. Cutaneous cryptococcosis in a donkey. Comp Clin Path 2006;15:271–3.
8. Powell RK, Bell NJ, Abreha T, et al. Cutaneous histoplasmosis in 13 Ethiopian donkeys. Vet Rec 2006;158:836–7.
9. Crothers S, White SD, Ihrke PJ, et al. Sporotrichosis: a retrospective evaluation of 23 cases seen in northern California (1987-2007). Vet Dermatol 2009;20: 249–59.
10. Fox R, Thiemann A, Everest D, et al. Molluscum contagiosum in two donkeys. Vet Rec 2012;170:649.
11. Davis WP, Peters DF, Dunstan RW. Besnoitiosis in a miniature donkey. Vet Dermatol 1997;8:139–43.
12. Dubey JP, Sreekumar C, Donovan T, et al. Redescription of *Besnoitia bennetti* (Protozoa: Apicomplexa) from the donkey (*Equus asinus*). Int J Parasitol 2005; 35:659–72.
13. Elsheikha HM, Mansfield LS, Morsy GH. Studies on *Besnoitiosis bennetti* in miniature donkeys. J Egypt Soc Parasitol 2008;38:171–84.
14. Ness SL, Peters-Kennedy J, Schares G, et al. Investigation of an outbreak of besnoitiosis in donkeys in northeastern Pennsylvania. J Am Vet Med Assoc 2012;240: 1329–37.
15. Elsheikha HM, Mackenzie CD, Rosenthal BM, et al. An outbreak of besnoitiosis in miniature donkeys. J Parasitol 2005;91:877–81.
16. Yeruham I, Braverman Y, Orgad U. Field observations in Israel on hypersensitivity in cattle, sheep and donkeys caused by *Culicoides*. Aust Vet J 1993;70:348–52.
17. Reid SW, Gettinby G, Fowler JN, et al. Epidemiological observations on sarcoids in a population of donkeys (*Equus asinus*). Vet Rec 1994;134:207–11.
18. Reid SW, Smith KT, Jarrett WF. Detection, cloning and characterisation of papillomaviral DNA present in sarcoid tumours of *Equus asinus*. Vet Rec 1994;135:430–2.
19. Nasir L, McFarlane ST, Torrontegui BO, et al. Screening for bovine papillomavirus in peripheral blood cells of donkeys with and without sarcoids. Res Vet Sci 1997; 63:89–90.
20. Bourdeau P, Baudry J. Pemphigus-type bullus dermatosis associated with pregnancy in a female donkey. Informations Dermatologiques Vétérinaires 2005;(11): 19–24 [in French].

21. Koutinas CK, Saridomichelakis MN, Mylonakis ME, et al. Equine hyperadrenocorticism: a report of 4 natural cases. J Hellenic Vet Med Soc 2004;55: 21–33.
22. Rickards K. Treatment of hyperadrenocorticism in donkeys. Vet Rec 2010; 166:152.
23. O' Grady SE. A fresh look at white line disease. Equine Vet Educ 2011;23:517–22.

Index

Note: Page numbers of article titles are in **boldface** type.

A

Adhesive tape impression + Diff Quik
    in EPD diagnosis, 583
Allergy(ies). *See also* Food allergy; *specific types, e.g., Culicoides* hypersensitivity
    treatment of, **551–557**
        atopic dermatitis, 554–555
        contact allergy, 555–556
        Culicoides hypersensitivity, 552–554
        food allergy, 555
        general concepts in, 551–552
        urticaria, 556
    update on, **541–550**
        atopic dermatitis–related, 546
        clinical disease expression–, diagnosis-, and treatment-related, 544
        food allergy, 546
        immunopathogenesis-related, 541–544
        insect bite hypersensitivity, 545–546
Alopecia(s), **629–641**. *See also specific types*
    alopecia areata, 630–636
    altered hair follicle function in, 636–639
    anagen effluvium, 637
    chemical toxicoses and, 639
    congenital, 640
    follicular dysplasia, 638–639
    hair follicle defects and, 639
    hair follicle inflammation and, 639–640
    hypothyroidism and, 637–638
    linear, 640
    noninflammatory, nonpruritic, **629–641**. *See also specific types, e.g.,* Alopecia areata
    seasonal, 637
    telogen effluvium, 636
Alopecia areata, 630–636
Anagen effluvium, 637
Antibiotic(s)
    in EPD management, 586
Antifungal agents
    in EPD management, 585
Antiparasitic therapy
    in EPD management, 586–587
Antiviral agents
    for sarcoid, 664

Vet Clin Equine 29 (2013) 709–716
http://dx.doi.org/10.1016/S0749-0739(13)00072-2
0749-0739/13/$ – see front matter © 2013 Elsevier Inc. All rights reserved.

vetequine.theclinics.com

Moving?

Make sure your subscription moves with you!

To notify us of your new address, find your **Clinics Account Number** (located on your mailing label above your name), and contact customer service at:

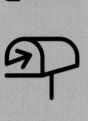

Email: journalscustomerservice-usa@elsevier.com

800-654-2452 (subscribers in the U.S. & Canada)
314-447-8871 (subscribers outside of the U.S. & Canada)

Fax number: 314-447-8029

Elsevier Health Sciences Division
Subscription Customer Service
3251 Riverport Lane
Maryland Heights, MO 63043

*To ensure uninterrupted delivery of your subscription, please notify us at least 4 weeks in advance of move.